Rosemary Gladstar's
Herbs *for*
REDUCING
STRESS &
ANXIETY

STOREY
BOOKS

*The mission of Storey Communications is to serve our customers
by publishing practical information that encourages
personal independence in harmony with the environment.*

This publication is intended to provide educational information for the reader on the covered subject. It is not intended to take the place of personalized medical counseling, diagnosis, and treatment from a trained health professional.

Edited by Deborah Balmuth and Robin Catalano
Cover design by Carol Jessop, Black Trout Design, and Meredith Maker
Back cover photograph by A. Blake Gardner
Cover and interior illustrations by Laura Tedeschi
Text design by Carol Jessop, Black Trout Design
Text production by Susan B. Bernier and Kelley Nesbit
Indexed by Nan Badgett, Word•a•bil•i•ty

Printed in Canada by Webcom Limited
10 9 8 7 6 5 4 3 2 1

Library of Congress Cataloging-in-Publication Data

Gladstar, Rosemary.
    [Herbs for reducing stress and axiety]
    Rosemary Gladstar's herbs for reducing stress and anxiety / Rosemary Gladstar.
        p.   cm.
    Includes bibliographical references and index.
    ISBN 1-58017-155-9 (pbk. : alk. paper)
    1. Stress management.   2. Herbs — Therapeutic use.   3. Materia Medica,
Vegetable.   I. Title.
    RA785.G59   1999
    615'.321—dc21   99-19491
                                                                          CIP

Dedication

My life centers around 500 acres on a mountaintop in the northeastern part of Vermont. There are endless helping hands that make it all possible: the gardens, the trails, the small orchard, the beehives, the woodlands, and the wildflower meadows. And the office that hums continuously, a hive of happy activity. There are a few people who never stop helping; they help with their hearts as well as their hands. This book is dedicated to them, the Sage Mountain staff: Robert Chartier, Katie Pickens, Nancy Scarzello, Karl Slick, Kathie Ross, Donna and David Bryant, and Matthais and Andrea Reisen.

Acknowledgments

I am sincerely indebted and grateful to the endless support and hard work of my editors, Robin Catalano and Deborah Balmuth. Their patience and caring sustained me through endless deadlines amid a schedule that was nothing less than chaotic. Due to their understanding, the help of the nervine herbs, and the view out my office window, I'm alive and well at the end of this writing odyssey.

CONTENTS

chapter one

Understanding the Nervous System

tress can be anything from the lash of a whip to a passionate kiss.

—Hans Selye

The nervous system (NS) is our link to our environment. It has three basic functions: to receive, to interpret, and to respond. Within the limited paradigm of modern Western science, this involves only our physical being and the physical world in which we live. We have our five basic senses to experience our external environment, and countless internal sensory neurons to monitor our internal environment. Then there are the some 12 billion cells that constitute our brain, the central computer or main station of the mind.

That alone would make the nervous system the most important system of our body. It is what provides integration and coordination to our lives. It allows us to see, feel, touch, act, and react. Without this basic physical NS response, there could be no life. To the degree that it is impaired, the quality, tone, color, and richness of life are diminished.

But the nervous system serves in a far greater capacity than just the physical quarterback of our body. It is that place where life itself, conscious self-awareness, attaches to the physical vehicle and converts the "puppet" into the "puppeteer." It is the interface where we can dream, think abstractly, create, and receive intuitive impressions. It is our primary connection to Universal Consciousness, or the divine in all of us.

The Final Frontier?

Western scientific culture and experimental techniques have shed great light on the workings of the human entity and the disease processes that affect it; however, there are many frontiers in medicine that continue to baffle the most ardent of researchers. As we discover more answers we are confronted with even more difficult questions.

The continuing exploration of the biological sciences provides us with the gross understanding of the human body and how it interacts with its environment. This progress has carried us to the exploration of ever more subtle areas of human metabolism. In these more elusive areas, the psychologist, the physicist, the microbiologist, the physiologist, the biochemist, and others must combine their thinking to push back the boundaries of our under-standing. The foremost physicists of the world are now adding the mystics and metaphysicians to their think tanks because particle physics has revealed that, no matter how much you dissect and reduce something, you can not get to an understanding of the whole by learning only about its tangible physical parts.

Interpreting the Signals

This, in part, is why the nervous system is such an excit-ing aspect of humankind. We can not understand conscious-ness or the interpretation of impulses by dissecting a brain. We can not understand how logical, rational thought occurs, or, even more baffling, how creative ideas spontaneously form in our minds.

Though it can be demonstrated which autonomic nerves control which involuntary body functions, what the neuro-chemical transmitters are and what their target sites are, and what part of the brain controls these processes, can anyone explain where the original awareness occurs that understands the need to send the message in the first place? And how does this awareness transform its desires or needs to the physical brain so the impulses can be sent?

We don't even really know what pain is, or why similar impulses can be interpreted as either pain or ecstasy. What hypotheses do we possess to define and explain emotions and feelings and where they originate and what effects they have on our systems?

Why does the heart keep beating and the breath continue to flow without our "conscious" intervention? And what causes them to eventually stop these functions, likewise without our apparent conscious intervention?

Asking the Right Questions

As much as we have learned about the nervous system, we are only scratching the surface. There comes a point where deductive and inductive reasoning and dissection arrive at an impasse. Without including the idea of a higher consciousness or higher order of the universe in their theoretical constructs, right-brain scientists are completely stymied at giving us answers to what many of us consider the *real* questions about life, how it works, and what its purpose may be.

With these thoughts in mind, it is important with the nervous system, perhaps more so than with any other system of the body, to address health and lack thereof from more than just a perspective of physical symptoms and treatments. Allopathic medicine, however appropriate for certain circumstances, treats NS disease primarily with drugs that interfere with or block the system's transmission and interpretation of impulses, or by surgical removal of unhealthy tissue. Considering how limited our knowledge in this field is, the irreversible nature of surgery should always be a last resort, after every other option has been explored.

STRESS IN THE MODERN WORLD

Svevo Brooks, author of *The Art of Good Living,* pinned down one of the Western world's largest problems when he observed, "As the pace of life quickens, we more deeply need calm, uninterrupted moments for the renewal they impart to our spirit. Leisurely walks, afternoon naps, the opportunity to stop and inhale the fragrance of a flower — these small interludes, once commonplace, are increasingly rare." Taking time for ourselves can do wonders for this most modern of problems.

Treating the Nervous System

The proprioceptive side of the nerves, the sensory receptors that respond to stimuli, is there to provide feedback to the brain and consciousness about vital body information. If we are suffering pain or distress, it is a warning of imbalance or danger to us. These warnings are only the *symptoms,* not the *originating causes.* If the smoke detector in your house goes off, the solution isn't to "deaden" it with a hammer. Wouldn't you be better advised to go look for a fire somewhere?

To continue the analogy further, it is often appropriate to shut off the alarm and stop the noise while searching for the source of the smoke. Allopathic medication often functions beautifully to alleviate acute pain. Unfortunately, for many, when the immediate pain subsides we forget to continue to "search for the fire."

Using Natural Therapies

The approach presented in this book is to provide tried-and-true ways to strengthen and build a healthy nervous system using natural therapies. Holistic treatments can be used in conjunction with conventional allopathic treatments to augment healing at all levels of life: physical, emotional, mental, and spiritual. In the great circle of holistic healing, all systems are part of the whole and should be used when appropriate.

The healthier the nervous system is, the better equipped to provide sensory input and motor response that facilitate optimum quality in our lives. Herbs and natural therapies play a vital role in the health and well-being of the nervous system. Not only are herbs full of concentrated nutrients that are important both nutritionally and medicinally, but herbs also form a direct link with intuition and higher intelligence.

Far more than just "green matter," herbs have an inherent ability to channel life energy and to connect with those places in us that are "disconnected" and in need of healing. Herbs

contain chemicals that have no apparent function for the life processes of the plant. However, these very chemicals have a direct and positive influence on the human body. Is there some divine plan at work here? Perhaps it is true that humankind's oldest system of medicine offers a form of healing that transcends the physical and connects us directly with a higher consciousness.

Reaping the Benefits

There are numerous physical ways that herbs benefit the nervous system. Because they serve as a source of energy and vitality for the entire body, herbs benefit the whole body while caring for the nervous system. Drinking a warm cup of chamomile tea after a long day at work is certainly a simple and rewarding way to relax the entire body. Immersing oneself in a warming, soothing bath in times of stress can be quite sustaining. Using herbs over an extended period of time for chronic stress problems can have long-term benefits. There are many excellent herbs and herbal formulas to use for relieving stress, anxiety, and mental tension.

Though herbs are not as effective as orthodox medicine in dealing with acute pain, they can help to relieve and soothe the pain through toning and nourishing the affected areas. Using herbs on a routine basis is a wonderful way to maintain a healthy, strong nervous system. In this way, herbs serve as preventive "medicine" — truly the best medicine of all.

ANCIENT WISDOM

The wise words of an ancient physician spoken in 1200 B.C. still apply: "First the word, then the plant, lastly the knife."

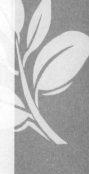

chapter two

Making and Using Herbal Remedies

T he quality of the herbs you use is important. Buy them from reputable dealers or, better yet, grow your own. Learn how to tell good-quality herbs by their color, taste, scent, and effect. If an herb is not effective it is probably because of either the quality or improper dosing.

Deciding the proper dosage of herbs for an individual is not an exact science. Even in conventional (allopathic) medicine, correct dosage is far more arbitrary than we're led to believe. Herbalists are just quicker to admit that determining the proper dosage for each individual involves some skill, a healthy touch of "inner knowing," observation, and a bit of guesswork.

Determining Dosage

I've found the guidelines in this chapter to be especially helpful for those just beginning their herbal studies. There are many considerations to take into account when determining proper dosage of an herbal preparation for the nervous system as well as for any other system of the body. One must consider the herb itself: what its primary action is, whether it has any toxic side effects, whether it's tonic in its action or is a specific medicine, and so on. One must also consider the constitution of the person: Is he or she relatively healthy? Robust or sensitive? Weak or debilitated? And, finally, one must consider the nature of the imbalance or illness: Is it chronic or acute? Excess or deficient in nature?

Taking these factors into account whenever possible will help you determine a more accurate dosage. Ultimately, when determining the correct amount of herbs to take, you must trust the wisdom of your own body; listen to what it's telling you, and ask the plants. They often give the best advice.

When unsure how much of an herbal preparation to take, use the following chart.

How to Determine Measurements

While many people are converting to the metric system, I've reverted to the Simpler's method of measuring. Many

Dosage Chart

Chronic problems *are long-term imbalances such as PMS, back pain, and insomnia. Chronic problems can flare up with acute symptoms, but the problem is long standing. Follow these guidelines when treating chronic problems:*

TEA	EXTRACTS/ TINCTURES*	CAPSULES/ TABLETS
3–4 cups daily for several weeks	½–1 teaspoon 3 times daily	2 capsules/ tablets 3 times daily

Acute problems *are sudden, reaching a crisis and needing immediate attention. Examples of acute problems include toothaches, headaches, migraines, menstrual cramps, and the pain caused by burns.*

TEA	EXTRACTS/ TINCTURES*	CAPSULES/ TABLETS
¼–½ cup throughout the day, up to 3–4 cups	¼–½ teaspoon every 30–60 minutes until symptoms subside	1 capsule/ tablet every hour until symptoms subside

includes syrups and elixirs

herbalists choose to use this system because it is extremely simple and very versatile. Throughout this book you'll see measurements referred to as "parts": 3 parts passionflower, 1 part lemon balm, 2 parts oat tops. The use of the word "part" allows the measurement to be determined in relation to the other ingredients. A part is a unit of measurement that can be interpreted to mean cups, ounces, pounds, tablespoons, or teaspoons — as long as you use that unit consistently throughout the recipe.

Sample Formula Blended in the Simpler's Method

PARTS	PARTS IN TABLESPOONS	PARTS IN TEASPOONS
3 parts passionflower	3 tablespoons passionflower	3 teaspoons passionflower
1 part lemon balm	1 tablespoon lemon balm	1 teaspoon lemon balm
2 parts oat tops	2 tablespoons oat tops	2 teaspoons oat tops

Medicinal Herb Tea

Herbs are available in many forms. The most common forms are tablets and capsules, tinctures, and the herb in its raw state for making tea. Tinctures and tablets/capsules are often preferred these days because of the ease in taking them. Though I appreciate these preparations, I prefer and recommend herb teas as part of every health regime. Why? Making herb teas helps us remain conscious of the essential part we play in our personal well-being. The mere act of preparing tea involves us in the healing process.

Tea is warming and soothing to our souls. It is as ancient as time itself and captures the essence of fire and water and plant life. When one brews a cup of tea, one performs an act of alchemy, the mixing and brewing of the elemental forces. Every health program should have as its foundation an herbal tea formula or two. You can add capsules and tinctures, herbal baths, or other treatments, but tea should be included as part of the program.

Method I: Infusion

Leaves, flowers, and aromatic plants require infusing or steeping as opposed to simmering because they lose their properties more quickly than do roots and barks. To make an infusion, boil one quart of water for each ounce of herb (or one cup of water to one tablespoon of herb), pour the water over the herbs and steep for 30 to 60 minutes. There are a hundred different proportions of water to herb and as many variations on the required time to infuse. Basically, every herb is different. Start out with the above recommendations and you'll soon get the hang of it. The more herb used and the longer it's steeped, the stronger the brew. Let your taste buds guide you.

Method II: Decoction

Decoctions are used with the more tenancious parts of the plant, such as roots, barks, and hard seeds or nuts. These plant materials require more direct heat and lower exposure to the heat. Place herbs in cold water, cover tightly, bring to a low simmer, and simmer for 30 to 45 minutes. Often, I'll let the herbs sit overnight in the water and strain the next morning.

Solar and Lunar Teas

I often use the energy of the sun and moon when preparing medicinal teas. Never underestimate the powers of these great luminaries; they affect us every day. Why not use that power to impact your tea? Solar energy is associated with masculine energy. I often make sun teas for people who are seeking to enhance the qualities of the sun in their lives: brightness, sunny disposition, largeness of spirit, warmth. The moon is the feminine luminary and is used to enhance dreams, visions, intuition, and the receptive part of oneself.

To make solar tea, place the herbs and water in a large jar with a tight-fitting lid. Place in direct sunlight and leave exposed to the sun for several hours. If you wish a particularly potent tea, prepare first as a standard infusion or decoction, and then offer the tea to the sun to work its magic.

To make lunar tea, place the herbs and water in a jar or glass bowl and place directly in the path of the moonlight. It's not important to place a lid on the container. Leave overnight and drink first thing in the morning. If you wish a particularly potent tea, prepare first as a standard infusion or decoction, then place the tea in the moonlight.

Capsules

Herbal capsules are one of the most popular ways to ingest herbs. They're quick and easy to take, as well as being virtually tasteless. But until recently, I didn't recommend capsules often because the herbs contained within them were usually less than poor quality. Herbs were typically ground with grinders that heated the plant material to more than 200 degrees, losing many of the vital constituents in the process. Most of the capsules used were gelatin based. These are difficult to digest and leave a gummy residue, not to mention they're a by-product of the slaughter industry.

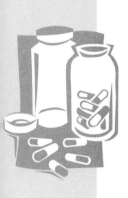

But there has been a transformation in the capsule industry. Veggie caps have recently become widely available. Plant based, these capsules dissolve quickly and are completely digestible. New cryogenic grinders powder the herbs at subzero temperatures, retaining all of the plant constituents. The powdered plants smell and taste fresh and are of far better quality. When buying capsules, buy from those companies that have gone to the extra trouble to ensure the quality of the product.

There are many ready-made herbal capsules on the market, but you can easily make your own. Although it is time consuming, it gives you control over which herbs you use and the quality of the product. Powdered herbs are simply placed in each side of a capsule, and the halves are joined. There are inexpensive machines available that quicken the job.

Powders

Powders are one of the easiest ways to take herbs, and can be used in far more creative ways than capsules. They can be added to food and drinks for a tasty and nutritious treat. Mix them into honey to form a paste. Try blending them in with blender drinks. Powders can also be combined with dried fruits, honey, and carob powder to make candy balls, a favorite herbal remedy for young and old alike. I especially like herbal powders added to soups and sprinkled in stir-fries. Be sure to purchase only good-quality herbal powders from reputable herb and natural foods stores, or grind your own.

Tinctures

Tinctures are concentrated extracts of herbs. They are taken simply by diluting a few drops of the tincture in warm water or juice. Most tinctures are made with alcohol as the primary solvent or extractant. Though the amount of alcohol is very small, many people choose not to use alcohol-based tinctures for a variety of sound reasons. You can also make effective tinctures with either vegetable glycerin or apple cider vinegar as the solvent. Though they may not be as strong as alcohol-based preparations, they are perfectly suited when alcohol is not tolerated.

Tinctures have a very long shelf life and should be stored in a cool, dark location. Because of their concentration, follow the dosage chart carefully.

Making Tinctures

There are several methods used to make tinctures. The traditional or Simpler's method is the one I prefer. It is an extremely simple system that produces beautiful tinctures every time. All that is required to make a tincture in the traditional method are the herbs, the menstruum (solvent), and a jar with a tight-fitting lid.

Step 1. Chop your herbs finely. I recommend using fresh herbs whenever possible. High-quality dried herbs will work well also, but one of the advantages of tincturing is the ability to preserve the fresh attributes of the plant.

Step 2. Place the herbs in a clean, dry jar. Pour the menstruum over the herbs. If using vegetable glycerin, dilute it with an equal amount of water. If using vinegar as the menstruum, warm it before pouring it over the herbs to help facilitate the release of herbal constituents. If choosing alcohol as your solvent, select one that is 80 to 100 proof, such as vodka, gin, or brandy. (Half of the "proof" of the alcohol is the percentage of alcohol in the spirits; 80 proof brandy contains 40 percent alcohol, 100 proof vodka contains 50 percent alcohol.) *Completely cover* the herbs with the menstruum and then add an additional two to three inches of liquid. Cover with a tight-fitting lid.

Step 3. Place the jar in a warm place and let the herbs and liquid soak (macerate) for four to six weeks. The longer the time, the better. I encourage the daily shaking of the bottles of tinctures during the maceration period. This not only prevents the herbs from packing down on the bottom of the jar, but is also an invitation for some of the old magic to come back into medicine making. Empower your herbal remedies with prayer and song.

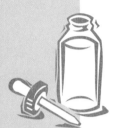

Step 4. Strain the herbs from the menstruum. Use a large stainless steel strainer lined with cheesecloth or muslin. Reserve the liquid, which is now a strong potent tincture, and compost the herbs. Rebottle and label.

Herbal Baths

Herbal baths are deeply relaxing. They help to take the edge off the day, calm and quiet the mind, encourage deep sleep, and sometimes are just the comfort one needs in a rough and busy world. Herbal bathing used to be far more popular than it is today. But as with so many other things in our busy lives, the quickness of showers has displaced the slow, peaceful nature of herbal bathing.

Making Herbal Baths

To make an herbal bath, use three to four ounces of herb per tub. Make a strong herbal tea and add to the bathwater, or tie the mixed herbs in a large cotton scarf and attach directly to the nozzle of the tub. Run hot water through the herbal bag until the tub is half filled, and then adjust the temperature with cold water. Soak in the bath for 20 to 30 minutes to enjoy the full benefits of the herbs.

Lavender oil is divine in the bath, creating a lasting relaxing feeling. When I travel, which I often do, lavender oil accompanies me like a steady friend. After a long day of traveling, it is a welcome addition to the bathwater and always, always, brings a sense of calm. See chapter 5 for herbal bath recipes.

chapter three

The Herbal Home
Medicine Chest

There are a number of remarkable herbs that reduce stress and anxiety, and directly benefit the nervous system. These herbs are generally referred to as herbal nervines. Unlike conventional medicines for NS disorders, which either deaden or nullify nerve response, nervine herbs are often toning and/or adaptogenic (helping the body adapt to stress) in action and have nutritive benefits for the nervous system.

Be Familiar with Nervine Categories

The following categories are helpful in defining the action of herbs on the nervous system. There is great overlap among these categories, but grouping the herbs gives some definition of how and what the herbs are doing in the body. Most herbal nervines do not manipulate life energy, but rather work in harmony with it. Those herbs strong enough to change energy patterns through manipulation are often the plant substances synthesized by drug companies and most are not legally available without prescription.

Nerve Tonics

Herbs that feed, tone, rehabilitate, and strengthen the nervous system are called nerve tonics. These herbs strengthen or fortify the nerve tissue directly and are generally high in calcium, magnesium, B vitamins, and protein. Though very effective, most are mild in action and can be taken over a long period of time. Herbs from this category are included in every formula for NS disorders.

Examples of nerve-tonic herbs are oatstraw, skullcap, wood betony, chamomile, valerian, hops, and lemon balm.

Nerve Sedatives

These herbs directly relax the nervous system and help reduce pain, ease tension, and encourage sleep. Unlike allopathic drugs, they do not accomplish this by deadening nerve endings, but rather by a gentle action that soothes and nourishes the peripheral nerves and muscle tissue.

Nerve sedatives include California poppy, passionflower, St.-John's-wort, catnip, valerian, lemon balm, hops, lobelia, skullcap, and cramp bark. Also included with the nerve sedatives are the antispasmodic herbs that help relieve muscle spasms and cramping.

Nervine Demulcents

These herbs are soothing and healing to irritated and inflamed nerve endings. The demulcent herbs have a gel-like consistency that coats and protects the nerve endings. Their actions are general and not specific to the nervous system, but they are included in almost all nervine formulas for their soothing, healing qualities and nutritional benefits.

Slippery elm bark, oats, barley, flaxseed, and marsh mallow root are all examples of nervine demulcents. Use only sustainably harvested slippery elm bark.

Nervine Stimulants

It is not often that stimulants, as we usually think of them, are recommended for NS disorders. When you are stressed, depressed, and worn out, the last thing you need is to have your system roused with caffeine-rich foods, sugar, or drugs — all common "remedies" for the blues. Instead, mild herbs that gently and surely nourish and spark the system are appropriate; they activate the nerve endings by increasing circulation, providing nutrients, and increasing vitality and zest. They neither provoke the system nor agitate it.

Try lemon balm, peppermint, ginkgo, gotu kola, spearmint, wintergreen, cayenne, ginger, bee pollen, eleutherococcus, ginseng, spirulina, rosemary, and sage if you need a stimulant.

Important Herbal Nervines

These herbs work by reconnecting the nerve channels in the body, gently stimulating or "reawakening" them. Rather than deadening pain, which most herbs can't do well, herbal nervines strengthen the nervous system so that it can better respond to pain. In essence, herbal nervine therapy increases our ability to cope with the daily stress of life.

Ashwangandha
(Withania somnifera)

Parts used: roots

Benefits: An ancient Ayurvedic herb, ashwangandha is referred to in India as the "Indian ginseng" and is used very much the way that ginseng is used in Asia. An excellent adaptogenic herb, ashwangandha increases the body's overall ability to deal with stress. It promotes general well-being and enhances stamina, thus its popularity with athletes. It is both energizing and soothing. Ashwangandha is primarily classified as a male tonic herb, though women use it as well. A classic reproductive tonic, it will help restore sexual "chi" or energy. It is specifically indicated for reduced levels of energy, general debilitation, reduced sexual energy, tension, stress, and anxiety. Especially useful for sexual problems associated with nervous stress.

Preparation tips: Said to have the smell of a female horse's urine and the stamina of a stallion, ashwangandha isn't the best-tasting herb, but it can be blended with other more flavorful herbs such as ginger, sarsaparilla, and cinnamon to make a suitable tasting tea. In India, the root is powdered and mixed with milk for a classic rejuvenating drink. Try blending it with your favorite chai blend, or try the tincture or capsule form.

California poppy (Eschscholzia californica)

Parts used: seeds, flowers, leaves

Benefits: This vibrant, golden blossom, California's state flower, grows in abundance in the United States. A kissing cousin of the notorious opium poppy, *Eschscholzia* has similar sedative and narcotic properties, but is much milder and nonaddictive. *Eschscholzia* is quite gentle in its action and is excellent in establishing equilibrium and calming nerve stress and excitability.

Suggested uses: The California poppy is especially recommended for children who have difficulty sleeping and who are overly excitable. Juliette de Bairacli Levy, the world-renowned herbalist and my mentor, suggests grinding the seeds into a meal and mixing them with honey. She dries these "cakes" in the sunlight to enhance their effects and then feeds them to children experiencing stress and anxiety.

Preparation tips: I suggest gathering the fresh plant just as the blossom opens. The seeds are best gathered after they are fully ripened and before the wind disperses them. To make a tea, pour one cup boiling water over one teaspoon of poppy seeds and blossoms, cover tightly, and let steep 20 minutes or overnight. Poppy can also be made into a tincture.

Catnip *(Nepeta cataria)*

Parts used: leaves, flowers

Benefits: This is another of those versatile wonder plants. Easy to grow, easy to prepare and use, catnip is safe as well as effective. A garden mint, it grows easily both in and out of the garden if you keep your cats away long enough for it to get a head start. While it sends cats into spasms of pleasure, it calms and sedates people, both young and old. It is especially valued as a safe, effective relaxant for babies and young children. Jethro Kloss, that famous old herbal doctor, writes in *Back to Eden,* "If every mother had catnip herb on the shelf, it would save her many a sleepless night and her child much suffering."

Suggested uses: An excellent calming herb, catnip can be used for all manner of stress. It is particularly beneficial for lowering fevers and for the pain of teething or toothaches. Serve as a tea throughout the day during teething pain. It is also a restorative digestive bitter and is used for indigestion, diarrhea, and colic. Give a couple drops of the tincture before meals to serve as a digestive aid. A few drops of the tincture before bedtime can help a fussy child sleep better. This is an excellent herb to help reduce fevers and can be used as both a tincture and an enema for this purpose.

Preparation tips: Catnip is quite bitter tasting, so it is often formulated with other more pleasant tasting herbs such as oats and lemon balm.

Chamomile (*Anthemis nobilis* and related species)

Parts used: primarily flowers, but leaves are useful

Benefits: One could not talk about the nervous system without mentioning chamomile. This is a small, beautiful, and gentle plant, long used as a beverage tea but equally valued for its powerful medicinal properties. Chamomile demonstrates to us that gentle does not mean less effective. It has been used for children's colic, nervous stress, infections, and stomach disorders. It is also highly effective against fever and inflammation. Remember the story of Peter Rabbit? When little Peter returned from Farmer John's garden — an extremely stressful experience considering he barely escaped with his life — his mother whipped him soundly, gave him a cup of chamomile tea, and sent him to bed.

Preparation tips: Pour one quart of boiling water over one ounce of chamomile flowers and steep, covered tightly, for 20 minutes. Drink three to four cups daily or as often as needed. This herb has lasting effects if used over a period of time. It is nice to blend with other nervine herbs, and is excellent for infants and children.

A VERSATILE PLANT

Pharmacological and clinical studies confirm what herbalists have long known; the common wayside plant known as chamomile is a very important medication for the nervous system. One of the major constituents of chamomile is a volatile oil obtained by steam distillation from the flower. The oil, which is a beautiful azure blue, is called azulen. Azulen contains a whole complex of active principles that serve as anti-inflammatory and antipyretic agents. The medicinal action of chamomile is most obvious in three major areas: the nervous system, the immune system, and the digestive system.

Feverfew (Chrysanthemum parthenium and Tanacetum parthenium)

Parts used: leaves, flowers

Benefits: Feverfew is another plant that has long been used by herbalists but virtually ignored by modern medicine. Recent pharmacological studies have proven its remarkable value in alleviating migraine headaches, inflammation, common headaches, and stress-related tension. Parthenolide, the active ingredient in feverfew, controls chemicals in the body responsible for producing allergic reactions and migraines. It also inhibits the production of prostaglandins that are implicated in inflammation, swelling, and PMS.

Suggested uses: Feverfew must be taken over a period of time to be effective. Though it will help to alleviate the pain of an active migraine, it is far more effective taken over a period of one to three months as a preventive. Its action is similar to aspirin, with a stronger but slower effect. Some people find that by eating a fresh leaf or two a day directly from the garden they are able to prevent migraines. Parthenolide is highly sensitive to heat and will be easily destroyed if feverfew is exposed to high heat in the drying or preparation process. If the product you are using is not effective, try another brand.

Caution: Feverfew can be taken over a long period of time by most people with no side effects; however, it does require some cautionary measures when used. Since one of feverfew's medicinal actions is to promote menstruation, it may stimulate the menstrual cycle unnecessarily or promote cramping and painful menstruation. It also is *not* recommended for pregnant women or for people taking anticoagulant drugs.

Preparation tips: I prefer blending feverfew with lavender and other nervine herbs for an effective remedy for migraine relief. Pour one quart boiling water over one ounce of feverfew flowers and leaves; add other desired herbs. Let steep 20 minutes, covered tightly. Strain and drink ¼ cup every half hour until the headache is gone. When using a tincture of feverfew, dilute ¼ teaspoon in ½ cup warm water or lemon balm tea every hour until the headache is cleared.

Ginkgo *(Ginkgo biloba)*

Parts used: leaves, fruits

Benefits: This is certainly one of my favorite herbs, and judging by the number of ginkgo products out there, a number of other people's as well. Though the fruits and seeds of ginkgo are considered of medicinal value, it is the fan-shaped leaves that are most often used. Historical evidence from China relating the use of the leaf to improve brain function is supported by more than forty years of clinical research in Europe.

Ginkgo works as a memory enhancer by increasing circulation and vasodilation in the cerebral region. Regular use of ginkgo improves mental stability and memory function, and increases mental vitality. It is also an excellent herb for vertigo and is an effective remedy for tinnitus, or ringing in the ear. It is one of the best circulatory herbs we have, promoting blood flow and oxygenation throughout the entire body. Ginkgo is an antioxidant and is useful against free radicals, substances that roam freely in the system, damaging cellular health and accelerating aging. I suggest this as a wonderful tonic herb for anyone over 45. You'll often find standardized ginkgo products on the market and I would recommend these as well as tea and whole plant tincture. I have seen ginkgo halt the progress of Alzheimer's and it may, in fact, be the most effective substance we have for slowing down this debilitating disease.

HERBAL HISTORY

Ginkgo is the sole remaining survivor of a large family of plants that date back several thousand years. In fact, there are fossil remains of ginkgo that date to the dinosaur era more than 200 million years ago. An excellent "brain food" and memory enhancer, perhaps ginkgo works in part because it holds the memories of an entire species — indeed, an entire age — in the cellular makeup of its being.

Suggested uses: To be effective, ginkgo must be used consistently for a period of two to four months. Though the effects of ginkgo are not sudden or dramatic, if taken over a period of time there is a noticeable increase of memory and vitality. Ginkgo works as a nutrient, not a drug, so it is necessary to be consistent and to use an adequate amount.

Preparation tips: Some studies suggest that ginkgo doesn't break down in water, but I have found it wonderfully effective as a tea. The ancients used it primarily in a water base, as well. As a tea for memory it blends well with sage, rosemary, and gotu kola. As a circulatory tea, blend it with hawthorn and lemon balm. For stress and anxiety, especially when it's mental worry, blend it with oats and nettle.

Ginseng, American *(Panax quinquefolius)*

Parts used: roots; should be at least five to six years old, the older the better.

Benefits: This is one of my favorite woodland plants, though it's difficult to find it in its native habitat these days. Connoisseurs of ginseng consider American ginseng the best in the world and Asian practitioners often prefer it. While Asian ginseng is warming and builds energy and heat in the body, *quinquefolius* is more neutral in its effects and tends to cool and soothe the system. It has the same tonic, adaptogenic effects as the Asian variety.

Suggested uses: Use for general debilitation, mental clarity, and nervous system toning. *Quinquefolius* is a balancing tonic for the entire body. It helps restore energy if used over a period of time. Used for anemia and other blood weaknesses. Good for exhaustion and for sexual dysfunction, especially when due to exhaustion or stress.

Caution: It is important to always verify where your roots are coming from. These plants are seriously at risk in their native habitat. Use only organically cultivated or woods-grown ginseng.

Preparation tips: Prepare the same as Asian ginseng. It has a wonderful bittersweet flavor and can be chewed.

Ginseng, Asian *(Panax* and related species)

Parts used: roots; should be at least five to six years old, the older the better

Benefits: Considered the "King of All Tonics," ginseng boasts one of the best reputations in the herbal kingdom. Its botanical name, *Panax,* means "cure-all" in Greek, and it has long been considered a male tonic herb. Often the older roots grow in the shape of men. Much of what is touted about ginseng is true, *if* you use good-quality, mature roots. Many of the roots and ginseng products sold on the market today are of inferior quality and have little therapeutic value. There are many varieties of *Panax* ginseng on the market (Asian, Korean, and Chinese); all varieties of ginseng are superior adaptogenic agents that help the body resist a wide spectrum of illnesses. When used over a period of time, ginseng revitalizes and restores energy and is especially good for building sexual vitality. Though most often associated with the male reproductive system, I've found ginseng to be equally good for women, especially women who need the "yang" (masculine) or grounding energy it's famous for.

Suggested uses: Ginseng rejuvenates the entire nervous system, regenerates frayed or overtaxed nerves, and discourages mood swings and depression. It restores sexual vitality and rebuilds and restores energy if used consistently.

Caution: Much of the Asian ginseng imported into this country and those Asian roots grown here are heavily sprayed with toxic substances. In one recent undercover operation, the USDA found more than 36 illegal toxic substances in roots harvested in Wisconsin. If the roots look large, overly plump, and whitish, be suspicious of the quality of the root. Buy only woods-grown or organically cultivated ginseng.

Preparation tips: Ginseng has a fine, robust flavor and makes a nice beverage tea. It blends well with many other tonic nervine herbs. I especially enjoy it served with ginger and cinnamon in a chai-type blend. Many people enjoy chewing on the pleasant tasting, bittersweet "sing root." Sliced and soaked in honey, it makes a tasty treat. Ginseng powder is also mixed with other tonic herbs and blended with honey

WHICH GINSENG SHOULD I USE?

I prefer the use of eleuthero to *Panax* varieties of ginseng, both because I find it works as well and because, unlike Asian and American varieties, it grows readily and in great abundance. Though not much eleuthero is cultivated in the United States, I've seen healthy specimens growing in parks and arboretums in the Northeast, suggesting that there are possibilities for commercial cultivation.

and spices to make a delicious concoction that can be used directly in tea or spread on crackers. Ginseng extracts and capsules are readily available, but because of its good flavor and ease of preparation, I suggest using it in powder form, cooking the roots in soups, and making tea with this granddaddy of all herbs.

Ginseng, Siberian (Eleutherococcus senticosus)

Parts used: roots, bark

Benefits: Siberian ginseng, also called eleuthero, has almost exactly the same properties as its cousin, *Panax* ginseng. It's a superior adaptogenic herb with an impressive range of health benefits. It is commonly used to increase stamina and endurance. It helps produce a state of nonspecific resistance against an underlying imbalance, regardless of the specific nature of the stressor. This is one of our best herbs for increasing endurance and stamina and for building and enhancing our resistance to stress factors, whether they are emotional, physical, or psychological. Siberian ginseng increases energy, and is used for suppressed sexual energy due to exhaustion and adrenal depletion.

Suggested uses: For best results, use over a period of time — several weeks to a few months.

Preparation tips: The flavor of eleuthero is rather inconspicuous and blends well with other tonic and adaptogenic herbs in tea. I also use the powder frequently in foods. The roots are an important ingredient in wines and elixirs.

Gotu kola *(Centella asiatica)*

Parts used: leaves

Benefits: This beautiful violetlike plant is native to tropical and subtropical regions of the world. It grows easily in the warmer areas of the United States or can be grown in greenhouses for a daily fresh supply of the tasty little leaves. It is especially recommended for memory loss. Considered one of the best nerve tonics, it has been used successfully in treatment programs for epilepsy, schizophrenic behavior, and Alzheimer's disease. Gotu kola is also an excellent stimulating nervine and is superb in formulas for nervous stress and debility. It gently but firmly increases mental alertness and vitality by feeding and nourishing the brain. Most of the gotu kola available commercially is of very poor quality. I recommend, if at all possible, growing this important herb or buying it from reliable sources. Buy only organically grown gotu kola; the commercial quality is unfit for human use.

Suggested uses: My favorite method for using gotu kola is as a tincture to strengthen memory function. It must be used consistently for at least four to six weeks before a difference is noticed. But don't expect to wake up one morning feeling like Einstein. Rather, you may experience a subtle but noticeable increase in memory and a pleasant feeling of being more mentally alert.

Preparation tips: Gotu kola is tasty and makes a lovely addition to teas. When fresh, it can be served raw as a salad green.

Hawthorn *(Crataegus* species)

Parts used: leaves, flowers, berries, tips of branches

Benefits: The flowers, berries, tips of branches, and leaves of hawthorn nourish, strengthen, and tone the heart muscle and its blood vessels. Though little is mentioned in literature, hawthorn is also a wonderful remedy for "broken hearts" and for depression and anxiety. It is a specific medicine for those who have a difficult time expressing their feelings or who suppress their emotions. Hawthorn helps the heart to flower, to open and be healed.

Suggested uses: This is a tonic herb and should be used over a period of time to be effective. Use in the form of tea, tincture, jam or jelly, and extract. Use hawthorn jam spread over crackers and toast to your heart's delight.

Caution: I have found hawthorn perfectly safe to use with heart medication, but if you decide to do so, you should consult with a holistic health care provider or a doctor knowledgeable about the use of herbs. Be sure that your practitioner is knowledgeable about both conventional (allopathic) medicine and alternative or complementary systems of healing.

Preparation tips: In Europe, where it's a revered and common medicine, hawthorn is prepared as jam. Hawthorn berry jam is delicious and readily available in grocery stores as well as pharmacies. Hawthorn berries also make a delicious tea and are often combined with lemon balm and oats for hypertension. The berries, leaves, and flowers are excellent combined with ginkgo leaves as a vascular tonic. For the treatment of high blood pressure, try combining hawthorn with yarrow and motherwort. Hawthorn is also effective in capsules, though it's so good tasting I would suggest more tasty herbal preparations when using it. It also makes a good tincture, but again the flavor can be utilized to make elixir and liqueur blends that are exquisite tasting and yet contain all of the nourishing benefits of the plant.

HERBAL HISTORY

The hawthorn tree was planted in or near most herb gardens throughout Europe and has been revered and surrounded by legend for centuries. When my grandmother came to this country, she planted hawthorns in the yard of each home she lived in. Many of those old hawthorns planted by her strong, worn hands still bloom.

Hops (Humulus lupulus)

Parts used: strobiles (the leaf bracts surrounding the tiny flowers), pollen

Benefits: Where I grew up in the beautiful
hills of northern California, the surrounding area was planted in hops. It is a beautiful
plant whose gold-dusted strobiles blossom in
the late summer and hang from a golden
green vine. It is these strobiles that contain the inconspicuous green flowers and the golden pollen grains that are the
medicinal parts of the plant. Rich in lupulin, volatile oils,
resins, and bitters, hops is a potent medicinal herb highly
valued for its sedative properties and relaxing effect on the
nervous system. It is especially useful for hypertension and
eases tension and anxiety. Hops is a powerful bitter, one of
our most potent, and is excellent as a digestive bitter. It's
especially useful for indigestion due to nervous energy and
anxiety, and is my favorite remedy for insomnia.

Suggested uses: For insomnia, I prefer a hops and valerian
tincture. Take a couple of hours before bedtime. Keep the
tincture bottle by the bedside. If you wake up in the middle
of the night, take several more large dropperfuls diluted in a
bit of warm water. As a digestive aid you can mix hops with
mugwort, motherwort, artichoke leaf, or any of the other
digestive bitters. Again, you may find this herb palatable
only if you tincture it. Take ½ teaspoon before meals.

Caution: Because it has such strong sedative properties,
hops is not recommended in large dosages for those suffering from depression.

Preparation tips: Hops is extremely bitter. Nothing really
disguises the taste well, so tea is not often recommended.
Generally, hops is tinctured or encapsulated. It is also a fine
medicine when made into beer and is quite sedative and
relaxing. Beer also serves as a milder form of hops as a
digestive bitter. Be sure the beer you drink is of high quality.
You can easily grow your own hops and make your own
home brew.

Kava kava (Piper methysticum)

Parts used: roots

Benefits: Kava is native to Polynesia, Melanesia, and Micronesia. Though highly revered for hundreds of years in its native culture, it hasn't been until fairly recently that kava became well known in the United States. In a few short years, it has climbed to the top of the chart in popularity. I have seen ads for it in newspapers, heard people talking about it in drugstores, and have been to more than one party where the beverage of choice has been kava. It truly is a remarkable herb and it's no wonder that it has gained such popularity here.

Kava has the unique ability to relax the body while awakening the mind. It produces a sense of relaxation and at the same time heightens awareness and makes you feel brighter. Primarily known for its relaxant properties, it helps reduce tension, anxiety, and stress. Its analgesic properties help alleviate pain. The kavalactones, active chemical compounds in kava, relax muscles rather than block neurotransmitters.

Suggested uses: Kava is available as tincture, extract, and capsules. The tincture is a quick, effective, and handy form to use. It is helpful in times of stress when you need a quick relaxant, something that helps put the world in perspective. Capsules are effective for long-term stress and anxiety.

Caution: Kava can be overused and abused. Though an herb of celebration, it was not meant to be drunk to the point of intoxication. It is a sacred herb in all the tribes that grow and use it, and is still used primarily in ceremonial fashion. Too much kava can make you nauseated, induce unconsciousness, and make you drive out of control. Be respectful of the power of this herb. Used judiciously, it is a wonderful relaxant and stress reliever.

Preparation tips: Kava has a unique flavor that may take getting used to. Don't be alarmed the first time you try it; it will numb the tongue and create tingling sensations throughout the mouth. These sensations are temporary and are caused by the kavalactones. There are very specific directions for preparing kava that many herbalists adhere to strictly. I generally prefer it as a tea or punch, and have found it to be very strong prepared this way, though a true kava connoisseur would snort at this method. Prepare a strong tea; add cinnamon, ginger, and cardamom for flavor. Let the tea sit overnight or several hours, then strain. Add pineapple juice and coconut milk for flavor and serve chilled. I've served this kava punch at large herbal functions. It definitely seems to elevate the spirits and brighten the mood.

Lemon balm (Melissa officinalis)

Parts used: leaves, flowers

Benefits: A fragrant and beautiful member of the mint family, *Melissa* not only is a gentle and effective nerve tonic but also tastes delicious. One can blend lemon balm with those not-so-pleasant-tasting nervines for a more drinkable blend. When crushed, the leaves of this plant smell like lemons. The leaves and flowers contain volatile oils, tannins, and bitters that have a definite relaxing effect on the stomach and nervous system. The medicinal effect of lemon balm is primarily sedative, relaxing, and mildly antispasmodic. It is excellent for stomach distress and general exhaustion.

Suggested uses: For a delicious nervine tonic, blend with chamomile and the milky green tops of oats.

Preparation tips: Pour one quart boiling water over one ounce of lemon balm. Let steep, covered tightly, for 20 minutes or overnight. Strain; drink four cups daily or as often as you need it.

Licorice (Glycyrrhiza glabra)

Parts used: roots

Benefits: This sweet root is an outstanding tonic herb for the endocrine system and is a specific for adrenal exhaustion, so prevalent in depression and lack of vitality. What is often classified as the midlife crisis may be closely or directly associated with adrenal exhaustion. Licorice supports the adrenals and will revitalize them if used over a period of weeks or months. Licorice is also highly regarded as a remedy for the respiratory system.

Suggested uses: Because of its extremely sweet flavor, licorice is best used with other herbs. For adrenal exhaustion, tiredness, and fatigue, drink two to three cups of licorice tea a day blended with wild yam, sarsaparilla, burdock root, and sassafras. Licorice is often made into cough syrups for sore throats, mixed with pleurisy root and elecampane for deep-seated bronchial inflammation, and combined with marsh mallow root for digestive inflammation and ulcers. Licorice can be used in tinctures and capsules, and because of both its flavor and its mucilaginous consistency, it's often blended in teas and cough syrups.

Caution: Although there are many warnings against using licorice, it must be remembered that licorice is one of the most widely prescribed herbs in the world; there are very few cases of toxicity reported due to its use. It is safe for children and the elderly, which generally means it's safe for everyone in between. It's particularly beneficial for those who suffer debilitating and wasting diseases. However, licorice is not recommended for individuals who have high blood pressure due to water retention. People who are on heart medication should check with their holistic health care providers before using licorice. There have been studies indicating licorice's ability to induce water retention and thus raise blood pressure levels, but most of the studies were done on licorice extracts, licorice candy, and allopathic medication — not on the whole plant or crude preparations made from licorice root.

Preparation tips: Because licorice is very sweet, it's often blended with other herbs to help flavor them. It is used in formulas to alleviate unpleasant symptoms caused by the action of harsher herbs without interfering with their beneficial qualities. It has a rich mucilaginous consistency and adds a soothing quality to any syrup or tea it's mixed with. I use licorice powder to flavor other herbal powders and then roll them into tasty little pills and balls.

Nettle *(Urtica dioica)*

Parts used: leaves, seeds, roots

Benefits: This is the stinging nettle that farmers despise, hikers hate, and children learn to deplore. But herbalists around the world fall at the feet of this "green goddess/man." What's so special about this prickly, somewhat incon- spicuous plant? It is a vitamin factory, rich in iron, calcium, potassium, silicon, magnesium, manganese, zinc, and chromium, as well as a host of other vitamins and minerals. It activates metabolism by strengthening and toning the entire system. It is a wonderful tonic for the endocrine and reproductive systems. It is indicated for liver problems and is excellent for allergies and hay fever. And because of its high calcium content, it is an excellent tonic for the nervous system. All this and it tastes good too.

Suggested uses: Nettle is most often served as tea, but it's delicious steamed and served as a green. Try it in place of spinach in spanikopita (Greek spinach pie) or with feta cheese and olive oil. You must make sure, however, that the nettle has been thoroughly cooked or you're likely to get pricked while eating it. For the nervous system it combines well as a tea with lemon balm, oats, and chamomile.

Preparation tips: Nettle has a rich green flavor and lends itself well to tea blends. I include it in many of my medicinal teas for the nervous system, reproductive system, liver, and urinary system. Combine it with green milky oat tops and raspberry leaf for reduced energy and sexual dysfunction. The tips of the nettle plant in early spring and summer are supe- rior, though I've eaten them throughout the season. If you have a good stand of nettles nearby, it is good practice to trim them constantly throughout the season. They will keep pro- ducing those tasty tops until fall. Ryan Drum, herbalist and wildcrafter extraordinaire, suggests the seeds are among the best and most nourishing of herbal stimulants. The roots traditionally have been steamed and eaten, though most people ignore them in favor of the tender tops.

Oats (*Avena sativa* [cultivated] and *A. fatua* [wild])

Parts used: green milky tops, seeds, stalks

Benefits: Oats are among the best of the tonic herbs used for the nervous system and are a superior cardiac tonic. Anyone who is overworked, stressed, or anxious, or who has irritated and inflamed nerve endings should include oats as part of a daily health program. Oats are one of the principal herbal aids used for convalescing after a long illness. They help soothe irritation from nicotine and other chemical withdrawals. Oats provide energy by increasing overall health and vitality. Oats are frequently used for NS disorders, depression and anxiety, low vitality, irritability, and urinary incontinence.

Suggested uses: Though the stalks are rich in silica and calcium, it is the fruit or seed that is primarily used for nerve disorders. The fruit contains several active alkaloids including trigonelline and gramine (found also in barley and passionflower), starch, and B vitamins. I recommend using the stalks and fruits together. They are at their best harvested when a green-gold, not fully ripe. Much of what is commercially available are the yellow stalks. Though this may be good for mulching the garden, it is not as good for medicinal tea. Look for the green-gold milky tops and stalks.

Preparation tips: We're used to thinking of oats in the classic form of oatmeal. But to herbalists, oatmeal is for breakfast, while oat tops are for tea. They are exceptionally rich in silica, calcium, and chromium and are one of the highest terrestrial sources of magnesium. The stalks of oats, though not as rich in minerals as the milky green tops, are also medicinal. Though many herbalists don't use the stalk, I've found they combine well with the upper part of the plant. Oats make a delicious, nutritive tea and can be combined with lemon balm and passionflower for a good nervine. Blend with valerian for a sleep aid. Combine oats with digestive bitters for any liver or digestive upset. And, finally, oats (both the meal and the unripened milky tops) make one of the most soothing herbal baths for nervous stress and irritated, itchy skin. Add several drops of lavender oil for an especially relaxing experience.

Passionflower (Passiflora incarnata)

Part used: leaves, flowers

Benefits: Contrary to what its name implies, passionflower is a calming, relaxing herb. Passionflower has a long history of use in its native land of South America, where it was used to treat epilepsy, anxiety, insomnia, and panic attacks. An effective but gentle herb, it can be used for hyperactive children as well as adults. Passionflower has some analgesic effects and is somewhat effective as a pain reliever for toothache, headache, and menstrual pain. It has strong antispasmodic actions, which make it useful for cramps and spastic or convulsive muscles.

Suggested uses: This plant is well known for its sleep-inducing properties and is often combined with valerian for this purpose. It is one of the best herbs for anxiety and depression and can be effectively combined with St.-John's-wort. Use the tincture at bedtime to aid in deep, restful sleep.

Preparation tips: Brew the leaves and flowers as an infusion and drink throughout the day.

HERBAL HISTORY

The name "passionflower" refers to the beautiful flower said to represent Christ's crucifixion: five stamens for the five wounds, three styles for the three nails, and white and purple-blue flowers representing purity and heaven. However, it is curious that this flower is native to South America, where the crucifixion story was unknown until the Spanish Inquistion. I've heard a story that a repenting Spanish priest seeking forgiveness from God after a particularly macabre massacre walked into the surrounding jungle. He found an exquisitely beautiful passionflower and took it as a sign of forgiveness.

St.-John's-wort *(Hypericum perforatum* and related species)

Parts used: leaves, flowers (approximately 70 percent flower to 30 percent leaf)

Benefits: This has become quite possibly the number one herb for depression and anxiety, the happy herb of the '90s. A classic herb for nerve damage and depression, St.-John's-wort has been used for centuries and has been held in high esteem by herbalists throughout Western Europe and the Mediterranean. It is primarily valued as an herbal remedy for damage to the nerve endings such as in burns, neuralgia, wounds, and trauma to the skin. It is also highly effective for stress, anxiety, depression, seasonal affective disorder, chronic fatigue, and personality disorders. It lifts the spirits and puts a bit of sunshine into the day. Early speculation targeted the plant as an MAO inhibitor, but this information has been rejected. In fact, the action of the plant is not fully understood, nor has the active chemical constituent responsible for its antidepressant activities been identified. Look to the whole wonder of this plant.

Suggested uses: Although St.-John's-wort is effective for depression, it is best used with holistic supportive therapies that include counseling, massage therapy, and foods specific for NS stress. St.-John's-wort combines well with other herbs and is often mixed with hops and valerian for insomnia, with lavender and lemon balm for depression, and with chamomile for children and young people going through emotional upheaval. I frequently combine it with passionflower *(Passaflora incarnata)* for anxiety and stress.

People often ask if taking St.-John's-wort is recommended while on prescription or over-the-counter antidepressants, with the hope of being able to decrease or eliminate those drugs altogether. Of course, it depends on the individual situation, but generally, if a person is not suicidal and doesn't have chronic clinical depression, I've found St.-John's-wort to serve very well as a transitional herb. Because one blocks the nerve responses and the other serves as a tonic building and strengthening aid to the nervous system, they don't interfere with their respective actions and create greater possibilities of healing when used together. It is important, however, when using these medications together, that one work closely with an experienced holistic practitioner.

Caution: St.-John's-wort does cause photosensitivy in some individuals. There was some earlier concern that St.-John's-wort worked similarly to Prozac as an MAO inhibitor, but studies have proven this theory to be false. Therefore, the restrictions imposed on MAO inhibiting antidepressants do not apply to St.-John's-wort.

Preparation tips: The beautiful red oil made magically from the cheerful yellow flowers is a wonderful "trauma" oil and is used for bruises, sprains, burns, and injuries of all kinds. It's a joy to behold and a joy to prepare. To make the oil, infuse freshly opened flowers in olive oil for two weeks.

Skullcap *(Scutellaria lateriflora)*

Parts used: leaves

Benefits: This beautiful, shy member of the mint family is found growing in shady areas near streams and meadows in the mountains. Somewhat inconspicuous, you may have to search to find it. Thankfully, it is readily available in most herb stores, as it is highly regarded for its nervine properties. Skullcap is one of the most versatile of the nervines and is indicated for all NS disorders, especially headaches, nerve tremors, stress, menstrual tension, insomnia, and nervous exhaustion.

Suggested uses: This is a strong, effective herb, and there is no danger of overdose or cumulative buildup if used over a long period of time. Quite the contrary; to receive the full benefit of skullcap it is recommended to use it over an extended period of time and in adequate dosages. Skullcap is used in tea, tincture, and capsule form. The suggested adult dose is two to three cups of tea daily or ¼ teaspoon tincture diluted in ½ cup warm water three times daily.

Preparation tips: For tea, use one teaspoon of the herb per cup of boiling water. Steep in water (do *not* boil the herb) for 20 minutes. Keep the lid on the pot while steeping.

Valerian (Valeriana officinalis and related species)

Parts used: roots

Benefits: One of the most potent herbs known for the nervous system, valerian is powerful, safe, and very effective. Scientific studies show that valerian works by depressing activity in the brain and spinal cord. It relaxes the smooth muscles of the uterus, colon, and bronchial passages. Valerian is the herb of choice by many people for stress, insomnia, and nervous system disorders. Though potent, it is perfectly safe to use and is not habit-forming. Valerian is effective both as a long-term nerve tonic and as a remedy for acute problems such as headaches and pain. It is one of the best herbs known for insomnia and restless sleep. Valerian has powerful tonic effects on the heart and is often recommended in combination with hawthorn berries for high blood pressure and irregular heartbeat.

Suggested uses: Some herbalists prefer the fresh, violet-scented roots; others claim the medicinal properties are stronger in the dried roots that smell like dirty socks. It's a personal preference, I've found. Though water soluble, most people don't prefer to take their valerian in tea form. It's usually taken either in tincture or capsule form. Don't be afraid to take adequate amounts of this herb. Begin with low dosages and increase until you feel its relaxing effects. If you take too much valerian, you might feel either a rubbery feeling in the muscles or a feeling of heaviness. Cut back the dosage so that you feel relaxed but alert.

Caution: Generally considered a safe, nontoxic herb, valerian can act as an irritant for some people. If you become further agitated and restless after using valerian, discontinue and consider yourself in that rare 5 percent of the population that shouldn't use this herb.

Preparation tips: Don't decoct these roots, as they are rich in aromatic oils. They should be infused only. Use one to two ounces of valerian root per quart of water. Pour boiling water over the root, cover tightly, and let the infusion sit overnight, or at least 45 minutes. Strain; drink four cups daily. If using a tincture, use one to two teaspoons diluted in warm water or tea three times daily or as often as needed. It is difficult, if not impossible, to mask the flavor of valerian. My suggestion is to just enjoy the strange flavor.

HERBAL HISTORY

Valerian has a long and colorful history and has been highly regarded as an herbal medicine for centuries. Hildegard von Bingen, a famous German abbess/herbalist, used it as a sedative in the twelfth century. In the 1500s medieval herbalist Gerard claimed it to be one of the most popular remedies of his time. Today valerian continues to be one of the most popular medicinal herbs in the world. In Europe it is used in hundreds of over-the-counter drugs and is relied on primarily as a medicine for stress and tension.

chapter four

Natural Remedies for Stress and Anxiety

The mind-body connection is one that is fraught with controversy and mystery. How do physical experiences affect the mind, and how do mental experiences influence the body? No one knows for sure yet, but we do know that a link between the mind and body exists.

Until recently, the majority of Western scientists were unwilling to recognize the connection between these two seemingly independent forces. But today, in the face of a host of modern depression-related disorders, people everywhere are turning to the natural world to heal themselves from the inside out.

Whatever your philosophy of life, the nervous system is your only means to connect and interact with your world. If you treat your nervous system like the sensitive instrument it is, it will play back the finest music to enrich your being. Keep it tuned and healthy, feed it well, and protect it from overuse and exploitation, and your rewards will be a life of exquisite quality. Through even the most stressful events, you will feel centered and empowered. Abuse it and the music turns to a cacophony of sound, the colors fade and run, the joy and zest for life drain away into indifference.

This chapter contains information on and remedies for common nervous system ailments. That part of you that can't be measured or quantified, that part that understands these words and makes rich associations from them, that part that can transcend all physical boundaries through the creative thought process is encompassed within the nervous system. The nervous system is your instrument of creation. You alone get to decide what kind of music you wish to play, what dance you wish to dance.

Anxiety, Stress, and Panic Attacks

We've all felt anxious at some time, overcome by anxiety at the thought of something fearful, either real or imagined. Talking in front of a group of people, a first date, a car coming at you on your side of the highway — these are all reasons for anxiety. Occasional apprehension is normal and sometimes the sanest response to a situation; frequent feelings of anxiety are not. The physical symptoms include accelerated heartbeat, rapid breathing, restlessness, and difficulty concentrating. Anxiety almost always precedes panic attacks. Living in a constant state of apprehension is a sign of major NS stress and should be attended to immediately.

Extreme, uncontrollable fear, often agoraphobic in nature, characterizes panic attacks. The fear frequently stems from unknown causes. Panic attacks may be a sane reaction to life in an insane world, the body's attempt to sound a loud, clear alarm. Unfortunately, panic attacks often do more harm than good to the person experiencing them, eroding his confidence, leaving him shaken and scared, and often with feelings of inadequacy and fear of recurrence.

Panic attacks tend to be preceded by periods of stress, insomnia, or poor dietary habits. It is essential when addressing a panic attack to seek out the reason behind it and work from there, correcting the underlying problem.

What to Do

Follow strict dietary guidelines for NS health. In anxiety, as important as what one eats is what one doesn't eat. Avoid all foods that irritate NS problems, especially stimulants. Concentrate on relaxing, nervine tonics and sedatives such as oat tops, lemon balm, California poppy, kava kava, and valerian. Drink three to four cups of relaxing tea a day. If feeling particularly apprehensive, take valerian tincture every hour until the anxiety subsides.

Flower essences are excellent for feelings of anxiety. See page 79 for descriptions of the various flower essences. If you find yourself feeling anxious, carry the designated flower essence for your particular problem with you at all times. Use it at the first sign of anxiety. For panic attacks, keep a bottle of Rescue Remedy on hand at all times.

Often high levels of noise or sudden movement agitate the sensation of fear and uncertainty. Avoid loud music and noises. Playing soothing music while in the tub drinking chamomile tea can often be the best remedy for the over-anxious individual.

Watch for symptoms of anxiousness in children and treat them with the same remedies and therapies as you would adults, but adjust the formulas accordingly. (See my book *Rosemary Gladstar's Herbal Remedies for Children's Health* for instructions on using herbs for children.) Herbs can also be used to relieve anxiety in animals. You may not be able to get your dog or cat to soak in a soothing bath, but you can give pets herb teas and flower essences, and alter their diets to include the foods that are helpful for anxiety. See C.J. Puotinen's excellent book *The Encyclopedia of Natural Pet Care* for more information on treating overanxious pets with herbs.

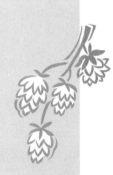

Hops Tincture

This tincture is an excellent remedy for nerve stress and debility.

> 2 ounces of high-quality hops strobiles
> brandy or vodka

1. Place the hops in a widemouthed quart jar. Add brandy or vodka to completely cover hops by 1–2 inches. Cover jar tightly and place in a warm (about 85°F), shaded area.
2. Let sit for 4–6 weeks, shaking occasionally to prevent the herb from settling on the bottom. Strain and rebottle for use. Take ½–1 teaspoonful 3 times a day.

Melissa Tea

Melissa, or lemon balm, is a wonderfully relaxing yet gently stimulating herb. It increases energy in the system by helping to release energy blocks and stress.

> 3 parts lemon balm
> 1 part lemon verbena
> 1 part chamomile
> 1 part St.-John's-wort
> 1 part borage flowers and leaves, if available

Combine herbs; prepare as an infusion, following the directions on page 10. Drink as often and as much as needed.

More Recommendations for Panic Attacks

From the treatments in both this section and Depression, choose a few suggestions that seem best suited for your situation. Because panic attacks are often about unconscious fears that are especially challenging to understand, it is often helpful to seek a counselor who is able to guide you on this journey. The best, most effective therapy I've found is Jungian Gestalt dream work and/or soul retrieval work. Plant spirit medicine, a shamanic herbal practice taught by well-known therapist Eliot Cowan, works with the spirit of the plant and is extremely effective for these types of situations. It may be difficult to find a practitioner, but it is well worth the effort. If interested in this type of herbal medicine, read Eliot's inspiring book *Plant Spirit Medicine.*

Chamomile Tisane

A relaxing, tasty evening drink, Chamomile Tisane gently soothes irritated nerve endings and eases away the day's tension.

> 4 parts chamomile blossoms
> 3 parts rose hips
> 2 parts lemon balm
> 1 part borage flowers and leaves, if available

Combine herbs; prepare as an infusion, following the directions on page 10. Drink as much and as often as needed. ❧

California Poppy Tea

This is a very soothing nervine tea, perfect for infants and children to help soothe the cares of the day.

> 1 part California poppy flowers and/or seeds
> 1 part chamomile
> 1 part oats, milky green tops
> ½ part marsh mallow root

Combine herbs. Following the directions on page 10, prepare as an infusion. Drink as much and as often as needed. ❧

Depression

Depression is characterized by extreme sadness, a sense of hopelessness and despair. It is caused by a variety of "lack factors," including lack of sleep, lack of nutrients, lack of light, and lack of love. Adrenal exhaustion, cold and damp conditions in the body, and hormonal and chemical imbalances can also contribute to depression.

What to Do

Sometimes depression is simply caused by a series of very sad, life-challenging or -threatening events. Like that smoke detector, depression is the symptom, not the cause, and is an indicator that things are awry. Fortunately, there are many treatments that can help alleviate depression.

Embrace life and love. The best thing we can do for ourselves during times of depression is to embrace ourselves, like a loving parent to a favorite child. Create love in your life, even love of gardening or hiking or sailing. It is essential to connect with nature during times of great depression. Find every reason you can to love yourself and everyone else. Generally, people who love others are loved by others.

Build and strengthen the nervous system so it can serve as the marvelous receptor and distributor of energy that it is. Follow all of the suggestions in chapter 5 that are appropriate to your situation. Concentrate on the herbs that are indicated for depression and sadness: St.-John's-wort, lemon

HEALING THROUGH READING

A good book to read during times of depression is Thomas Moore's *Care of the Soul*. Though certainly not a book about depression, it is in essence a guide on how to live soulfully in a troubled world, and it's soul food for a troubled spirit. But don't limit yourself to just one book; read any kind of literature that lifts your spirits and soothes your soul.

balm, oats, and lavender. Emphasize a diet high in calcium and B vitamin–rich foods. Review the list of nervines included in chapter 3 and incorporate all that feel right to you. Drink three cups daily of High Calcium Tea (page 63), Nerve Formula for Depression (below), or Nerve Tonic Formula (page 64).

Use flower essences; they are strongly indicated for depression and go straight to the issues, even when you're uncertain what they are. Find a flower essence practitioner in your area and make an appointment for a consultation, or use one of the excellent books that guides you, step-by-step, through how to select the appropriate flower essence. See page 79 for a list of flower essences most often recommended for NS disorders.

Take evening baths of lavender and lemon balm. If you have a garden, collect roses and borage flowers and add them to the bath. This isn't a treatment only for women; men will benefit from it just as much. Herbal bathing can be soothing to a weary soul. You might even consider installing an outdoor tub in your garden. It's a bit hard to remain depressed for long while soaking in a flower-strewn tub surrounded by plants in the garden. However short, this respite from the cares of the world is welcome relief.

Incorporate different forms of massage into your routine. Sometimes, treating yourself from the outside in helps heal the source of the problem.

Listen to your dreams. Often, it is in the dreams that the answers come. Our primal consciousness speaks to us in the dark shadows of the night.

Nerve Formula for Depression

> 2 parts chamomile
> 1 part borage flowers, if available
> ½ part lavender flowers
> ½ part roses
> 1 part lemon balm

Mix herbs. Make an infusion following the directions on page 10. Drink 1 cup 3 times a day. 🌿

Headache

Considered the most common affliction of humankind, in the United States alone more than a half-billion dollars are spent yearly on headache medication. Headaches are the result of a number of different problems, including low blood sugar, constipation, toxicity of the blood, allergies, lack of sleep, eye stress, mental stress, and emotional tension. In rare cases headaches can signal deeper problems, such as brain tumors, but most often headaches are the body's complaint against the overtaxed mind. Though there are hundreds of drugs promising instant headache cures, the cause of the headache has to be corrected before the problem is solved.

Excluding migraines, headaches basically fall into two categories: vascular headaches, which are caused by dilation of the blood vessels in the head, and tension headaches, which are caused by constriction or tension of the muscles in the scalp, neck, and head.

Nerve Formula for Headaches

3 parts lemon balm
3 parts chamomile
1 part skullcap
1 part passionflower

Combine herbs; prepare as an infusion as instructed on page 10. Drink ½ cup every hour until symptoms subside.

Treating Vascular Headaches

Vascular headaches are generally the result of too much cold food in the diet and an overly acidic condition of the body. Foods such as ice cream, cold liquids, alcohol, and sweets can agitate the vascular type of headache.

Quickly alkalize the diet with salty, contractive foods such as Umeboshi plums (available in natural foods and Asian grocery stores), brined cured olives, and a strong alkalizing tea blend. Vascular headaches respond to proper treatment within 15 to 60 minutes.

Alkalizing Herb Blend for Vascular Headaches

    1 part yellow dock root
    3 parts dandelion root
    2 parts burdock root
    skullcap or valerian tincture

Decoct the roots as instructed on page 9. Drink ¼ cup of tea every half hour until symptoms subside. Add ¼ teaspoon skullcap tincture or ¼ teaspoon valerian tincture to each cup of tea for best effect. 🌿

Treating Tension Headaches

Tension headaches are usually the result of stress, tension, heat, lack of fluids or food, low blood sugar, salty foods, or excess mental concentration. The next time you get a headache, try to identify the foods you ate or the activity you engaged in prior to the onset of symptoms. This will help you determine the best treatment.

Tension headaches may take a longer time than vascular headaches to respond to treatment, sometimes up to 24 hours. Remedies consist of balancing the contractive condition of the body with cooling liquids and foods, and foods that are sweet or sour. These include apple juice with lemon, unsweetened cranberry juice, applesauce with lemon juice, and room-temperature herbal teas such as chamomile and lemon balm served with lemon.

Other Treatments

Recurring headaches indicate that there are deeper issues that need addressing. Look first at lifestyle. Allergies can also be a reason for recurring headaches. Are you eating foods that might trigger a chemical reaction in your system? Do you have allergies to pollen, mold, grass, or other natural substances? Poor digestion or intestinal infection can cause headaches in susceptible individuals. Is your diet good? Do you have regular bowel movements? Is your food digested well? If a headache persists or if you have recurring headaches, consult a holistic or medical practitioner.

The following suggestions are effective, safe treatments for both vascular and tension headaches.

- Hot herbal footbaths are wonderful remedies for headaches. See page 73 for a good recipe. While soaking your feet in the hot herbal water, place a cold ice pack over the forehead or nape of neck. The cold will *not* cause more muscle tension in the case of tension headache. Drink a warm nervine tea such as a skullcap–feverfew–chamomile blend.
- Valerian tincture — ¼ teaspoon diluted in warm chamomile tea or water — can be taken every half hour until the headache is gone.
- Feverfew–Lavender Tea should be drunk in frequent ¼ cup doses until the headache is gone. Follow the instructions on page 50, using 3 parts feverfew and 1 part lavender. Make a quart at a time.
- Niacinamide has been very effective for many people suffering from headaches. Take 100 mg of this B vitamin three times daily.
- Changing your activity is one of the most effective home treatments for tension headaches. If the headache comes after driving for several hours, sitting at a desk, at a meeting, or any other sedentary activity, switch to something more active. Take a brisk walk, jog, or find some other form of vigorous physical activity.

Skullcap Tea

Skullcap is a wonderful herb for treating headaches and nervous stress.

    2 parts skullcap
    2 parts lemon balm
    1 part feverfew
    1 part chamomile

Combine herbs; prepare as an infusion as instructed on page 10. Drink at least ¼ cup every half hour until the headache symptoms are gone. ✺

Migraine Headaches

Migraines are similar to tension headaches in that they are contractive in nature and caused by similar imbalances, but they are far more severe and are often recurring. Consequently, they are more difficult to correct. Migraines are a signal from the body to the brain that it's reached its limit; they are often experienced by people who expect much of themselves.

Nutrition, or lack of it, plays a major role in both the occurrence and treatment of migraines. Allergic reactions to certain foods often trigger a migraine. The offending foods may not be linked to the migraine because symptoms generally do not arise for several hours. Follow the dietary suggestions listed for tension headaches. Migraines have been linked to genetic components, but more often are the result of allergies, tension, immune suppression, or a combination of all these factors.

What to Do

Though there are several classifications of migraines, the symptoms and causes are similar and the treatment is much the same. Many of the drugs available for migraines are considered to have harmful side effects and, though they offer temporary relief, none will cure the condition. Migraines are generally corrected only after a long and serious commitment to alter lifestyle patterns that contribute to the problem. Incorporating many of the suggestions listed for tension headaches (see page 47) and those in chapter 5 will be helpful, along with these treatments.

At the first signs of a migraine, begin taking niacinamide, 300 mg daily; vitamin B$_6$, 200 mg daily; and rutin, 200 ml daily. Divide the doses and take two or three times during the day. Alacer's Emergen-C is also very effective in helping to prevent migraines when taken at the onset of the symptoms. Take two packages (2,000 ml) of Emergen-C twice a day.

Some types of migraines respond remarkably well to a potent dose of coffee or other caffeine-rich herbs. In tension headaches, the veins contract and pressure builds in the head; caffeine quickly dilates the capillaries, initiating a sudden burst of blood through the veins. I have seen this very powerful remedy work several times.

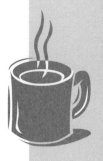

Feverfew for Migraines

Feverfew is the herbal medicine with the greatest success rate for migraine sufferers. It is not a "quick fix"; it is more effective as a preventive than as a curative for the active stages of the migraine. Many people report good results using the tincture or tea, as well as eating one or two fresh leaves daily. It must be used over an extended period of time to be effective, and the quality of the herb must be good. Feverfew does not normally have side effects, but pregnant women should not use it. If you are a menstruating woman and experience cramps or excessive bleeding while using feverfew, discontinue its use.

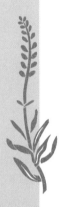

Feverfew–Lavender Tea or Tincture for Headaches

> 2 parts feverfew blossoms
> 1 part peppermint
> ½ part lavender blossoms

1. Combine herbs. To prepare as an infusion, follow the directions on page 10. Drink ¼ cup every half hour until headache symptoms have passed.
2. To make a tincture, follow the directions on page 13. Take ¼ teaspoon of the tincture 3 times daily.

CONNECTING WITH NATURE DURING STRESS

"We need the tonic of the wilderness," said Henry David Thoreau. The ocean, the mountains, the deserts, a wooded grove — all contain the "magic" needed to restore pure radiant energy to a stressed soul. The Mother Earth in all of her infinite compassion and strength has remarkable powers to restore vitality. Wash yourself in the pure water of the streams, put your bare feet on the good earth, fall asleep in the arms of an ancient tree. There is good medicine to be found in nature. It is long lasting and heals the soul.

Jethro Kloss's Famous Antispasmodic Tincture

This formula is a favorite remedy of Jethro Kloss, a famous herbal doctor of the early 1900s.

1 part lobelia seed or leaf
1 part skullcap leaf
1 part myrrh resin
1 part skunk cabbage leaf
1 part black cohosh root
1 part valerian root
¼ part cayenne
brandy or vodka (80 proof)

1. Combine herbs. Place the mixture in a widemouthed quart jar. Add brandy or vodka until the herbs are covered by an inch or two of the alcohol. Put a tight-fitting lid on the jar and place in a warm, shaded area for 4–6 weeks. Shake occasionally to prevent herbs from settling on the bottom.
2. Strain and rebottle the liquid for use. Take ¼ teaspoon of the tincture diluted in warm water or tea every half hour or more often until symptoms subside. 🌿

Herpes

A painful viral infection that can reside dormant on the nerve endings for many years, herpes has increased in such epidemic proportions that it has become the second most common venereal disease in the United States. Both herpes simplex II, genital herpes, and herpes simplex I, a less painful though even more common type of herpes that appears as cold sores and fever blisters, are agitated by stress, tension, a compromised immune system, and a sugar-rich diet. Holistic treatment of the nervous system has successfully eliminated many cases and offers not only temporary relief from the virus but lasting results. The following suggestions are also useful in treating shingles or herpes zoster, an even more painful type of herpes that most often afflicts the elderly.

Preventive Measures

Avoid all sugars and sweet foods, especially chocolate. Herpes thrives on a sugar-rich, acidic system. Also avoid foods high in arginine, an amino acid that is found in excessive amounts in people who have herpes. Foods high in arginine include peanuts, peanut butter, and chocolate. Include foods in the diet that are rich in calcium and B vitamins. Yogurt, kefir, nutritional yeast, spirulina, and miso are exceptional foods for people experiencing herpes. See other dietary suggestions in chapter 5.

Follow the suggestions in chapter 5 for supporting the nervous system. In addition, take echinacea tincture (¼ teaspoon two to three times a day, five days of the week) for three months to build and strengthen immune health. I prefer blending echinacea with astragalus as a tonic immune-enchancer. Whenever you experience even the first signs of a herpes outbreak, take ¼ teaspoon of the tincture every hour.

Drink several cups a day of bitter teas that are liver cooling, such as Oregon grape root, dandelion root, and yellow dock root. They will help fight off the infection and alkalize the system. If feelings of depression are overcoming you, reach for St.-John's-wort. It is a worthy friend at such times and has antiviral activities as well.

Supplement your diet with 500 mg of L-Lysine daily for three months. Some people have experienced excellent results from taking high doses of L-Lysine until symptoms have subsided. The suggested amount is 2,000 mg three times daily. Do not continue this dosage for extended periods of time.

Reishi, matiake, and shiitake mushrooms are all indicated for viral infections and help support the function of the immune system. Though the names may appear unfamiliar to

SIMPLE WISDOM

Sometimes all that it takes to make a miracle is a warm cup of chamomile tea and a hug.

— Dr. Tieraona Lowdog

you, these mushrooms are, in fact, commonly used. Shiitake, a delicious and tender morsel, should be used as food on a weekly basis. Reishi and matiake are most often taken in tincture form, though they can be cooked in soup and served several times during the week.

"Quick Fixes"

It is possible to recognize a herpes outbreak before the lesions appear. There are definite signals your body relays to you. Pay attention to your body and listen to its signals. For external relief of herpes symptoms, the following suggestions have all proven helpful. Different cases respond to different treatments, so experiment until you find the one that brings the most relief.

- Licorice root extract applied topically to the lesions is the most effective remedy I know of. Keep a bottle handy and apply at the moment you feel an outbreak occurring. It is effective on both cold sores and genital herpes. Apply several times daily.
- Another effective treatment is essential oil of lemon balm. Used throughout Europe to treat herpes outbreaks, it is not so well known in the United States, but people have reported excellent results. Apply several times daily.
- Aloe vera gel brings a cooling relief and helps to gently dry up the herpes blisters. Apply several times daily.
- Combine green volcanic clay, organically cultivated goldenseal or Chinese coptis, and myrrh powder. Mix into a paste with water or aloe vera gel and spread over the blisters.
- An herbal salve made with St.-John's-wort, comfrey, and calendula is wonderfully soothing and healing. You can puchase this salve ready-made or make your own.
- A mixture of yogurt and acidophilus applied to genital blisters will help heal them, although it may sting a bit at first.

Insomnia

One out of three Americans suffers from insomnia at some time. Purportedly caused by stress, anxiety, depression, and physiological disorders, insomnia aggravates and is aggravated by nervous system disorders. Though the body needs only a couple of hours of rest to recharge its battery, the brain and nervous system suffer without the necessary six to eight hours of sleep a night.

What to Do

If you are suffering from insomnia, these steps almost always remedy the problem. But insomnia is only a symptom of an imbalance. It is important to look at the greater picture and correct the cause.

Step 1. Beginning four hours before bedtime, take valerian/skullcap tincture, ¼ teaspoon every hour.

Step 2. Four hours before bedtime take a high calcium/magnesium formula or High Calcium Tea (see page 63 for recipe).

Step 3. Right before bedtime drink a warm cup of milk (or soy, almond, or rice milk) with cinnamon and honey added. These milks, unlike cow's milk, do not have high amounts of L-tryptophan, but they are both tasty and very soothing.

Step 4. Keep valerian/skullcap tincture by your bedside. Take ½ to 1 teaspoon as needed.

Step 5. If you do wake up, which you may, do not try to force yourself back to sleep. That is an exhausting process and seldom works. Instead, keep a boring book by your bedside and read. Or, draw a hot herbal bath and soak for a half hour or so. Sip a strong nervine tea while soaking.

Step 6. If experiencing a long-term period of insomnia, follow the suggestions in chapter 5 for building the nervous system. Include massage, hand- and footbaths, lavender oil baths, and daily exercise.

Step 7. About 20 minutes before bedtime, take a brisk walk or go jogging. If possible, walk barefoot for a time to connect with the Earth. For many people, brisk physical exercise relaxes and nourishes the nervous system and allows a deep, relaxed sleep.

Sleep Pillow

One of my favorite ways to use hops is to sew them into sleep or dream pillows. These recipes trace back hundreds of years. The lavender oil enhances the herbs' relaxing effects. For vivid dreams, add an equal amount of mugwort to the blend.

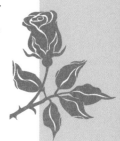

- 1 part dried hops
- 1 part dried roses
- 1 part dried chamomile
- 1 part dried lavender
- 1–2 drops lavender oil

Mix herbs. Stuff a small pillow with the herb mixture. Sleep with it tucked into your pillowcase, close to your head.

Nerve Formula for Insomnia

This blend is extremely effective if taken in frequent doses before bedtime. It will be quite bitter due to the hops; you may wish to tincture it, in which case increase the amount of hops and valerian.

- ½ part hops
- 1 part valerian
- 3 parts chamomile
- 1 part oats
- 1 part passionflower

Combine herbs. Follow instructions for making an infusion on page 10. Take small, frequent doses of the formula about 3 hours before bedtime.

DEVELOPING AWARENESS

Temporary insomnia can be used as a tool to develop psychic awareness. Those unusual waking hours are an excellent time to write in your journal, pray, and do "inner" work that is difficult to find time for during the day. If insomnia persists, however, it will wear down the psyche, as rest is essential to the health of the nervous system.

Neuralgia/Pain

Pain is the result, not the cause, of illness. It is the sensation or feeling that the body sends to the brain that signals something is awry. Though the underlying problem ultimately needs to be corrected, the very nature of pain calls for immediate attention.

What to Do

Allopathic medicine certainly offers a wide selection of effective medications that provide quick pain relief. When instant pain relief is needed, these medications are superior to herbal remedies. Though sometimes necessary, these medications work by tampering with the signals of the nervous system. Often pain is manageable, and is a valuable part of the healing process.

At times it may be necessary to utilize the quick-acting pain-relieving drugs, but they are overused and often abused in our society. The following suggestions offer reliable *alternatives.* Although these herbs are most often used for mild to moderate pain, they can be effective for severe pain when the dosage and frequency of use are increased.

St.-John's-wort oil and St.-John's-wort tincture work effectively for relieving pain. Use the oil externally and the tincture internally, several times daily or as often as needed.

Valerian tincture is an effective pain reliever and has special benefits for pain of the muscles and skeletal structure. Take the tincture frequently until the pain subsides. I have given large doses of the tincture successfully for severe pain caused by second-degree burns. Within 15 minutes the pain was bearable, though it might have helped that the valerian was in a base of high-quality brandy!

Herbs high in salicylic acid, such as willow bark, wintergreen, and meadowsweet (*Spiraea* species) have been used for centuries to relieve the pain of inflammation and fevers. These herbs were the original active ingredients in aspirin.

Herbal nervines (see page 17) are effective for relief of pain and should be given in small, frequent doses. For instance, when administering a tincture give ¼ teaspoon every 15 to 30 minutes until the pain subsides.

California poppy, though nowhere near as strong as its exotic Oriental cousin, the opium poppy, nonetheless has effective pain-relieving properties. It is effective for inducing sleep and helping to reduce pain.

St.-John's-Wort Oil

This oil is generally used topically for nerve damage, pain, swellings, bruises, and other types of trauma to the skin. But I like to use St.-John's-wort internally as well. I add it to salad dressings and mix it in with stir-fries. I even mix it with my animals' food when they are particularly stressed or anxious.

Collect St.-John's-wort blossoms just as they are opening. Pinch a bud and a squirt of bloodlike oil should burst out. If ready, the buds will stain your fingers bright red. Traditionally, people collected the herb on the anniversary of the day St. John the Baptist was beheaded.

Although the flowers are preferred, some leaves are useful; I generally suggest roughly 70 percent flowers to 30 percent leaves. The ripening of the buds depends on weather conditions and location. Allow the buds to air dry in a warm, shaded area for a few hours. Though this isn't always necessary, it allows some of the moisture to evaporate and, most importantly, it's a polite way to let whatever tiny creatures have made their home in the flowers an opportunity to escape.

> St.-John's-wort flowers and leaves
> virgin olive oil

1. Place the herbs in a widemouthed jar and cover with 2–3 inches of high-quality olive oil. Cover tightly and place the jar in a warm, sunny location for 4–6 weeks.

2. Strain the oil through a fine meshed strainer and rebottle. The oil should be a deep blood red, the redder the better. Apply topically to sprains, bruises, wounds, swellings, and other areas of tissue trauma.

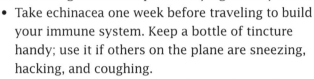

Tips for Stressless Traveling

Traveling, often a wonderfully exciting experience, can also be extremely stressful, especially when it involves flying. Flying subjects the body to added stress and recycled air, and it upsets our natural rhythms by interfering with our biological time clocks. People who fly often find themselves with compromised immune systems and are often more prone to illness. Following are some tips for staying healthy in the air:

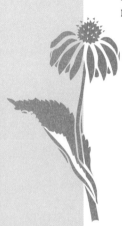

- Take echinacea one week before traveling to build your immune system. Keep a bottle of tincture handy; use it if others on the plane are sneezing, hacking, and coughing.
- Kava kava is the flyer's friend. It can help take the anxiety out of the most stressful situation. When things get boring, it can spice up the atmosphere a bit. It's especially useful for nervous situations such as delayed flights, engines that don't start, and turbulence.
- Rescue Remedy is the traveler's "first-aid kit." Use for stressful or traumatic situations. It's tasteless, very effective, and safe to use with any other type of medication.
- Ginger is good for motion sickness and nausea. My mentor, Juliette de Bairacli Levy, always travels with ginger candy for stomach disorders. The problem for me is that it's too good and often gets eaten as a snack!
- It is essential to drink extra water when flying. I usually pack a quart bottle of my own. It's added weight, and water is served on the plane, but I prefer drinking my own fresh mountain water from home.
- For jet lag, take ginkgo–hawthorn tincture. Begin taking it a couple days before flying.
- Melatonin is an excellent remedy for jet lag and in almost all cases will eliminate it. Take ½ to 1 mg of melatonin before flying.
- Pack a half-ounce bottle of essential oil of lavender. Virtually first aid in a bottle, I use a few drops of the lavender oil as a perfume for deep relaxation.

HOW DO I PACK ALL THIS?

Does it seem that there's no room left in my suitcase for anything else? Actually, I pack my herbal treatments in a small cosmetic bag. It amounts to three bottles of tincture (kava kava, schizandra–Siberian ginseng, and echinacea), a small bag of powdered ginger, half-ounce bottles of Rescue Remedy and lavender essential oil, a small container of melatonin, and several packages of Emergen-C. The only bulky items are the water and spritzer bottles. Have I ever gotten sick from all the flying I do? Only once. I had some unexplainable stomach pains that were, I'm convinced, from butterflies in my stomach because I was going to see my honey.

- Adaptogenic herbs can help relieve the stress of traveling. My favorite tincture combination is schizandra berries and Siberian ginseng. Take this combination before traveling and have it on hand during the trip as well. You can use ½ to 1 teaspoonful of the tincture 3 times a day, or as needed.
- A small spritzer bottle filled with fresh water, essential oil of lavender, and a drop or two of Rescue Remedy is the perfect remedy for stale airplane air. Check with your seatmate before misting the air.
- Finally, I always travel with Alacer's Emergen-C. I find this particular brand of vitamin C to be particularly helpful for eliminating jet lag, warding off sickness, and for bursts of energy when needed. Two at a time is recommended.

Withdrawal

Addiction is both a physiological and physical dependency on a substance. Food, sugar, prescription drugs, recreational drugs, tobacco, and coffee are all common substances of addiction. You can even become addicted to a lack of food. Addictions can be difficult to break; in fact, for many people they are the most difficult challenge they will ever have to face.

We often think of cocaine, speed, and alcohol when we think of addictive substances and we think of those "others" who are addicted. In treatment centers for illicit and prescription drug addictions, the most difficult "drugs" for addicts to give up are coffee and tobacco, our socially endorsed drugs of choice for the 20th century. Often, addicts are counseled not to give these up, because they are inexpensive, readily available, and socially acceptable. They serve as a permissable crutch for the addictive personality. However, each of these substances has serious repercussions when consumed in any more than moderate amounts.

Tobacco, long touted as a "cool" thing is a powerful carcinogen. Furthermore, the chemicals used to grow it spread toxic substances in the environment. Coffee, a wonderful, benevolent substance when consumed in modest amounts, is highly addictive — try going without it for a day or two. Daily use in many individuals will cause severe depletion of the adrenals and constant agitation of the nervous system. Sugar, a highly addictive, refined substance, is known to create health problems and increase tooth decay, obesity, and personality disorders. None of these substances is bad in and of itself; in fact, each is a special substance used in ceremonies and rituals by various cultures. But overconsumption causes health problems and addictions.

What to Do

Herbal nervines, adaptogenic herbs, and blood cleansers or alteratives are the herbal groups that most benefit the addict. My close friend and fellow herbalist Jean Argus started her successful tea company, Jean's Green, with an herbal detox formula she developed at the request of her brother, who worked as an acupuncturist in a drug rehabilitation ward of a large hospital. De-Tox Tea, the formula Jean created both to cleanse the body and to eliminate the desire for the addictive substance, has remained her best-selling tea and is available in several hospital wards where addictions are treated. (See Resources for more information on Jean's Greens.)

Herbs especially recommended during drug withdrawals include:

- Milk thistle seed. This excellent herb is one of the few substances known that will actually rebuild damaged liver tissue. It is excellent for drug withdrawals, to cleanse the liver, and to help repair damage to the liver due to excess alcohol and other types of drugs, including prescription medications. Milk thistle can be taken as a liquid extract, a standardized preparation, and in capsules. To make tea, grind seeds first.
- St.-John's-wort. Probably the number one herbal treatment for depression and stress, St.-John's-wort aids in stabilizing mood swings associated with drug withdrawal.
- Red clover. One of the best blood cleansers or detoxifiers, red clover has been used extensively in detox formulas.
- Burdock. The root and seeds of burdock are excellent for liver support and detoxification.
- Goldenseal and Chinese coptis. For liver inflammation and congestion, these two herbs are excellent. They will stimulate liver and gallbladder function, which is essential to cleansing the system. Use these plants only if they are organically grown.
- Valerian. When experiencing withdrawal symptoms, use valerian to help relax muscles and reduce pain.
- Oats. Use the milky tops for agitated and irritated nerves. The soothing, nourishing properties of oats make them one of the best nutritive aids for the stress of withdrawal symptoms.
- Astragalus. A superior adaptogenic herb, astragalus tones and strengthens the entire system.
- Echinacea. The body goes through tremendous internal stress when "forsaking" an addiction, making you susceptible to illness and physical challenge. Echinacea fortifies the system.
- Essiac. Not an herb but a formula, Essiac is a simple, effective cleansing tea that lessons the symptoms of all types of drug withdrawal.

Most people associate caffeine with coffee, but other foods such as guarana, chocolate, and kola nuts also contain this substance; avoid these foods if you are trying to cut down on your caffeine intake. To help you get through caffeine withdrawal, first cut your regular coffee consumption by half. Substitute the missing coffee with herb teas or grain beverage blends such as Cafex and Postum. A spicy chai blend can also help wean you off coffee.

If you're quitting cigarette smoking, take ½ teaspoon of red clover tincture three times daily to help cleanse the body of nicotine. Two cups of milk thistle seed tea taken three times daily will help detoxify the liver.

Excellent Herbal Formulas for the Nervous System

The following herbal formulas are among my favorites for the nervous system. Some of the formulas are calming or pain relieving. Others supply a spark to gently energize. But all of the herbs included here provide nutrients that help strengthen and support this marvelous system.

Ginkgo Leaf Tea

For increased memory, emotional stability, and energy, try this formula.

>   2 parts ginkgo leaf
>   1 part gotu kola
>   1 part peppermint

Combine herbs. Follow instructions on page 10 for making an infusion, and drink 3–4 cups daily for 3 months. In order for ginkgo to be effective, it must be used with some consistency. I suggest taking it for 5 days, resting for 2, and repeating this cycle for 3–4 months.

Brain Tonic Tincture

I call this recipe Memory Lane. It's often the first tincture I teach my students how to make. It calms and strengthens the nervous system and increases memory. It must be used consistently for at least 4–6 weeks before a difference is noticed.

    2 parts gotu kola
    2 parts ginkgo leaf
    1 part peppermint
    ½ part sage
    ½ part rosemary
    brandy or vodka (80 proof)

Place herbs in a widemouthed jar and cover with brandy or vodka. Cover the jar with a tight-fitting lid and place in a warm, shaded area for 6–8 weeks. Shake the bottle every few days to prevent the herbs from settling on the bottom. Strain and rebottle for use. Recommended daily dose: ½–1 teaspoon of tincture diluted in ¼ cup warm water, juice, or tea 2 times daily for 2–3 months.

High Calcium Tea

This tea is meant to be used over a 3- to 4-month period. By supplying calcium, it provides a calming action to the nervous system.

    1 part oats and oatstraw
    1 part nettle
    1 part horsetail (shave grass)

Combine herbs. Prepare as an infusion as directed on page 10. Drink 3–4 cups daily.

Valerian Tea

A hearty, relaxing blend, Valerian Tea is one of the better-tasting valerian blends.

½ part licorice root
1 part valerian root
2 parts lemon balm

Following the instructions on page 11, decoct the licorice root for 15 minutes. Turn off the heat and add the valerian root and lemon balm. Infuse for 45 minutes. Strain; drink as much and as often as needed.

Nerve Tonic Formula #1

Drink this general rejuvenator for the nervous system daily for 2–3 months. Feel the stress just slip away.

1 part chamomile
3 parts lemon balm
1 part oats
½ part chrysanthemum flowers
¼ part lavender flowers
½ part rose petals
stevia to taste (optional)

Combine herbs. Follow instructions on page 10 for making an infusion. Drink 1 cup 3–4 times daily.

Nerve Tonic Formula #2

This is a very energizing and revitalizing root blend. Most of the herbs are easily obtained in herb stores.

½ part ginseng root, sliced
1 part licorice root
2 parts eleutherococcus (Siberian ginseng)
1 part astragalus
1 part cinnamon
½ part ginger
½ part cardamom seeds
2 parts dandelion root
1 part burdock root

Combine herbs. Prepare as a decotion, following the instructions on page 11. Drink 1 cup 3 times a day.

chapter five

Promoting Well-Being from Within

This chapter contains suggestions to help build and strengthen the nervous system. They can be used in conjunction with other forms of treatments, such as allopathic medication or combined with systems of natural medicine to create a holistic treatment plan for building strength and vitality.

As with most forms of natural healing, *consistency* is the key to health and well-being. Herbs and natural remedies will not always alleviate pain and nervous stress as quickly as allopathic drugs that are designed to quickly and effectively deaden our senses. Natural therapies will, when used over an extended period of time, rebuild the nerve connections and create a lasting flow of vibrant energy. Most natural therapies for NS disorders are based on nutrition, herbs, exercise, and a reevaluation of lifestyle.

Use Nutrition as a Pathway to Health

Dietary imbalances and unhealthy eating patterns contribute to many of the problems of NS disorders, especially those associated with stress and anxiety. Likewise, a well-balanced diet will support and build a healthy nervous system. Because whole foods are not vitamin and mineral pills, they contain all the necessary nutrients needed to be properly assimilated and utilized by your body. While excellent therapeutics and fine for remedying problems, vitamin and mineral supplements do not provide the whole spectrum of nutrients, and certainly don't provide them in a manner that our bodies have been evolving with and utilizing for many centuries.

There is an ongoing debate among nutritionists concerning the inability to obtain all of our nutrients from food. This is a sad argument at best. Organic agriculture based on sustainable, renewable practices replenishes both the earth and our bodies and provides high-quality food rich in the total spectrum of nutrients. If we insist on eating demineralized processed food, then yes, the chances of getting necessary nutrients is highly questionable. If one further argues that organic food is priced beyond the average person, check out the price of vitamin and mineral supplements. What you save on supplementing your diet with these pills can buy a lot of organic food. But everyone, even those with the smallest garden space, can grow an organic vegetable garden. Aside from high-quality organic food and the satisfaction of restoring the earth, gardening is simply one of the best therapies for stress and anxiety.

Make a checklist of these whole food "supplements" and see how many are included on a regular basis in your diet. If they are found lacking, you may wish to include them daily for proper NS functioning. A diet specific to NS health should emphasize alkalizing foods such as fresh sprouts, high-quality protein, whole grains, green leafy vegetables, root vegetables, cultured milk products (such as yogurt, kefir, and buttermilk), lemons and grapefruit, and seeds and nuts.

The following are suggestions for food sources that contain the essential vitamins and minerals specifically needed for the health of the nervous system.

Calcium

Calcium is well known for its role in building strong bones and teeth. Its role in the health of the nervous system is not as well known, yet it is essential for healthy nerve function. Proper amounts of blood calcium prevent nervousness, irritability, muscle spasms, muscle cramping, hyperactivity, and insomnia. Fortunately, calcium is abundant in our diets and is found in easily digestible forms in seaweed, yogurt and other milk products, and most dark green leafy vegetables such as spinach, chard, broccoli, turnip greens, kale, beet greens, and parsley. It is also found in high amounts in almonds and sesame seeds. Though milk is touted as a high source of calcium it is, in fact, sorely lacking in the amounts and type needed by our bodies.

Seaweeds are particularly high in calcium. A major food source in many parts of the world, seaweed is often neglected as a high-calcium food in American diets. For comparison, 3½ ounces of cow's milk contains 118 mg of calcium. The same amount of hizike (a mild-flavored seaweed) contains 1,400 mg. Kelp contains 1,093 mg, and wakame contains 1,300 mg.

Along with foods high in calcium, you may wish to add a calcium supplement to your diet during times of high stress, anxiety, or when working on NS disorders. If using pills, be certain the calcium is from an organic source and is bio-chelated for easier assimilation.

There are many herbs that provide high-quality calcium. These include:

- Oats
- Nettle
- Dandelion greens
- Mustard greens
- Horsetail
- Chickweed
- Amaranth
- Watercress

B Vitamins Are Essential for Mental Health

The B vitamin complex comprises 11 essential vitamins. All are dependent on one another and are essential for mental health, a well-balanced nervous system, and healthy metabolism. When symptoms of mental distress or disorders such as irritability, nervousness, panic attacks, excess fear, depression, or suicidal tendencies appear, this is often an indication of B vitamin deficiency.

Though each B vitamin has a specific role in the physiology of the body and psychology of the mind, they are synergistic with one another. An excess of one of the B vitamins for a long period of time will, sooner or later, result in a deficiency of the others. B vitamins are most effective taken as a complex. For NS disorders look for those foods that are especially high in pantothenic acid (B_5) and pyridoxine (B_6).

Vitamin B_5 is the most important of the B vitamins for relieving stress. Vitamin B_6, together with vitamin C, helps to form the brain chemical serotonin, which promotes calm moods and deep sleep. (Another important factor for normal serotonin levels is getting enough sleep. People who are sleep deprived often suffer from low serotonin levels, resulting in anxiety, stress and mental distress.)

The B vitamins are found in high concentrations in dark green leafy vegetables, whole grains, whole wheat, brown rice, oatmeal, yogurt, kefir, wheat germ, molasses, and dried beans. Nuts and seeds are also generally high in B vitamins. Some of the highest sources of B vitamins are nutritional yeast, spirulina, and bee pollen.

Herbs high in B vitamins include:
- Parsley
- Dandelion greens
- Nettle
- Sesame seeds
- Seaweeds
- Wild oats

The Wonder of Spirulina

Spirulina is a blue-green algae that grows on freshwater ponds. Respected as an excellent source of nutrition in many cultures for centuries, it only found its way into the American diet a decade or two ago, and only in a limited manner. Its use is primarily restricted to those who shop in natural foods stores. Too bad, as it could benefit so many!

An excellent nutrient for the nervous systesm, spirulina is rich in B vitamins and gammalinolenic acid (GLA), which helps reduce inflammation, and, thus, reduces irritation. It contains 60 to 70 percent protein by weight, second only to dried whole eggs as a source of protein. People often complain about the flavor of spirulina, but it is far better than dried eggs!

Spirulina is available in tablets and powder form. I recommend the powder for quality and economy, but most people find the "green" taste and looks overpowering and opt for the tablets. A recommended amount would be two tablespoons of the powder or six to ten tablets daily. Though people sometimes balk at the high price, it is quite economical when purchased by the pound. It can be purchased in bulk from Frontier Herbs or Trinity Herb Company at very reasonable prices (see Resources).

Bee Pollen: A Powerhouse of Energy

This potent, magical food made from the flowers is the designer food of the bees. A concentrated form of nearly all known nutrients, bee pollen provides a powerhouse of energy for the nervous system. A complete protein containing all 22 amino acids, bee pollen has a higher concentration of the eight essential amino acids (those not produced in our bodies) than most other forms of protein. In addition to its protein content, bee pollen contains high levels of 27 different minerals, enzymes, and coenzymes, vitamins B_1, B_2, B_6, niacin, pantothenic acid, folic acid, vitamin C, and the fat-soluble vitamins A and E.

A combined miracle of flowers and bees, these tiny grains of pollen provide some of nature's finest nutrition. A wonderfully uplifting food, bee pollen captures the essence of flowers and the energy of bees and transforms that energy into food for our human nervous system. A small amount during times of stress often works wonders.

Use only small amounts, out of respect for the energy that the bees put into collecting these golden grains of pollen. It is recommended to eat no more than one to two teaspoons a day and never waste a kernel — each teaspoon contains 4.8 billion grains of pollen! For the best quality, use fresh pollen, not tablets. Always eat it raw — sprinkled over salads, in yogurt, by itself, or in blender drinks.

Some people suffer allergic reactions to bee pollen; others claim it helps clear their allergies. The first time you try some, take just a few grains to test for allergic reactions.

Add Nutritional Yeast to Your Diet

Nutritional yeast, commonly referred to as brewer's yeast, is a superior source of protein and includes all of the essential amino acids. It provides therapeutic benefits for most NS disorders. Along with its 50 percent protein content, nutritional yeast is also one of the best sources of the entire B vitamin complex (excluding B_{12}). Nutritional yeast is also an excellent source of many minerals and trace elements, including selenium, chromium, iron, potassium, and

YEAST AND BEER?

In spite of its nutritional credentials, many people shy away from eating nutritional yeast because of the flavor. Originally a by-product of the beer-making industry, this microscopic plant organism, *Saccharomyces cerevisiae*, was grown in vats containing grain, malt, and hops. Yeast took on the characteristic bitter flavor of the hops. Most yeast on the market today, however, does not come from breweries. It is grown on various media, including molasses, sugar beets, whey, and wood sugar for the purpose of being sold as nutritional supplements, and the flavor has greatly improved.

phosphorus, and is extraordinarily rich in nucleic acids, including RNA factors.

Yeast comes in powders, flakes, and tablets. The powder is the most potent, the flakes dissolve easier and often taste the best, and the tablets are the least effective and most costly. Cooking with it will destroy some of the B vitamins and nutrients, so it is best to eat it in its raw state. Mix with juices and blender drinks, sprinkle on vegetables, salads, and popcorn. There are numerous creative ways you can find to enjoy this potent, vitamin-laden little substance. *Note:* Nutritional yeast is *not* baker's yeast.

When I first began using nutritional yeast 25 years ago, there was only one kind available, the by-product of the breweries, and it was bitter. But I have always appreciated its high nutritional content and found ways to enjoy it in tomato juice, with cottage cheese, and in soups and salads. Today, many of the flavors of the nutritional yeast are quite good and actually enjoyable. To help your taste buds adjust to the flavor, start by taking small amounts of nutritional yeast (one teaspoon twice a day) and work up to one to two tablespoons. It is good in protein shakes, salads, casseroles, and soups.

If you are depleted in B vitamins, nutritional yeast may at first cause gas and bloating if too much is taken at once; experiment with small amounts until you find the nutritional yeast that works best for you. People who suffer from yeast infections *(Candida albicans)* should not eat yeast or fermented foods, as it may agitate the yeast infection. I have not found this to be the case, but it is the current popular opinion and I will respectfully pass it on.

Natural Therapies for Nervous System Health

We all yearn to feel balanced, in harmony, at peace with our environment, but we often are distracted by the chaotic nature of the world we live in and then expect a "quick ride" back to our place of center, of calm. There are ways to be fully present and involved in the chaos of the world, but still remain calm, centered, and at peace with your inner environment.

I have found that even in the busiest of lifestyles it is easy to maintain that sense of center we long for, but it requires basic commonsense practices and a maintenance program to sustain that feeling. Knowing what the connection is between our nervous system and our environment is helpful; knowing what foods feed and build our nervous system is also helpful. Equally important is being conscious of what creates for us as individuals that feeling of calm in the eye of the hurricane.

Lots of natural therapies support NS health and vitality. Combined with herbs, diet, and whole food supplements, these simple practices will help guide you to that perfect place of calm. They are especially useful combined with other therapies for NS disorders.

Energize with an Herbal Footbath

For many people, stress focuses in their heads. It gets stuck, so to speak, in the mental plane. This is perhaps why stress so often results in headaches and mental disorders. Though hot herbal footbaths feel great any time, they are especially recommended for headaches and mental stress.

HEALING WITH NATURE

When I wash my face in the sink, splash water from a fountain, take a bath, I am always reminded of the stream or river or ocean that these drops of water flow from.

— Svevo Brooks

They are deeply relaxing, easy to do, and are an excellent way to relieve head tension and stress.

This headache/stress treatment takes more time and energy than swallowing an aspirin, but the results will be deeply satisfying and long lasting.

Herbal Footbath

You may, of course, use any combination of relaxing herbs you have at hand. Mustard powder, ginger, sage, and rosemary are all good herbs for footbaths. Quaker Oats are excellent, also, and will do in a pinch.

> 2 parts lavender
> 1 part hops
> 1 part sage
> ½ part rosemary
> a few drops lavender oil (optional)

1. Place herbs in a large pot and fill with water. Place a lid on tightly and bring to a low simmer. Simmer over low heat for 5–10 minutes. Pour into a large basin and adjust temperature with cold water. It is important to keep the footbath water *very* hot. It should be hot enough to be almost uncomfortable but without burning the feet.

2. Make yourself comfortable in the softest, coziest chair you have. Slowly immerse feet in the water. Cover the basin with a thick towel to keep the heat in. It helps to have a friend massage your feet, head, and shoulders. Refill the basin with hot herbal tea as it cools. Play quiet, relaxing music in the background or listen to the silence. While bathing your feet, sip a cup of chamomile or feverfew–lavender tea.

Relax in an Herbal Bath

To make an herbal bath, follow the same instructions given for footbaths, but increase the amount of herbs that is used. I generally suggest three to four ounces of herb per tub. Lavender oil enhances the calming effects of the bath.

Herbal Bath

> 2 parts lavender
> 1 part hops
> 1 part sage
> ½ part rosemary
> a few drops lavender oil (optional)

Make a strong herbal tea and add the water to the tub, tie the herbs in a large cotton scarf and attach directly to the nozzle of the tub. Run hot water through the herbal bag until the tub is half filled, and then adjust the temperature with cold water.

Massage

People have found relief from stress and tension in the many forms of massage therapy offered today. Because we recognize that much of the psychological tension and stress of the nervous system is held in the physical body, gentle manipulation of the muscles that hold that tension is often extremely helpful. A well-trained massage practitioner not only has the ability to work out present tension, but also is able to train the body to release tension as it builds.

Many people consider massage an unaffordable luxury, but in times of nervous stress and life upheavals it is often a valuable and necessary therapeutic technique. There are many systems of massage, from gentle Esalen/Swedish-style massage to deep tissue work. Like most therapies, you may have to experiment and research the various systems before deciding which form works best for you.

Massage is among my favorite methods of relieving stress. It works for muscle stress as well as stress held deep in the inner recesses of the body. Often trauma, fear, panic attacks, and severe depression respond to the touch of a skilled body worker. Painful memories can become reasons for stress and physical pain as much as actual injury. Massage helps not only with the physical symptoms, but with the internal programming as well. It is important to find a good massage practitioner and to decide on a form of massage that is most suitable for your own particular type of stress.

I was in a fairly bad car accident several months ago and though the three of us in the car were basically unharmed, the car rolled several times. The only injury was to my shoulder, but at the time it seemed hardly worth mentioning. We declined a ride in the ambulance to the local hospital, took a little Rescue Remedy, and decided a soak at a local hot tub was the remedy needed to wash our aches and fears away.

Several weeks later my shoulder began aching severely, as much from the stress of the accident, I think, as the injury to the muscle. I tried stretching, resting, moving, and holding it, and finally called my favorite masseuses, Matthais and Andrea Reisen. Body workers for many years, these two expert therapists specialize in cranial sacral massage, a form of body work that moves energy through the body and helps unlock old memories and patterns experienced as blockages. Three sessions of cranial sacral work later — without the use of body touching — my shoulder no longer held on to the trauma and was able to release whatever residual pain remained.

Exercise

Physical exercise is one of the best methods we have available to release the stress and tension of our minds and our bodies. Like massage therapy and bathing, exercise helps move the disorders and tension of the mind into physical matter, and from the physical body it is better able to release it as energy into the universe.

Exercise assures a good flow of blood to all parts of the body. It helps move us out of our heads, where so much of our stress is stuck. Exercise is a valuable part of any therapy for NS disorders. When you find yourself facing life changes, upheavals, or are under stress, be absolutely sure you increase your exercise accordingly.

REAPING THE BENEFITS OF OUTDOOR EXERCISE

When I was going through the upheaval of divorce several years ago, I took up running. I always ran on the same woodland path, as the familiarity of it gave me some reassurance. Along with the physical benefits of running, I began to notice how much quieter my mind felt after the run. But the greatest benefit was making all those friends en route. I would pass the same plants, the same grand trees. I would stop each day and talk to a huge old yellow birch, telling it my troubles and how I was doing that day. Exercised helped, but Nature, my running partner, helped even more.

There are so many forms of exercise available today, from outdoor sports to TV aerobics, from yoga and gentle stretching to weight lifting at the local gym. There are suitable exercise programs for every body type, age, and condition. Your responsibility is to find the type most suitable for your personal needs and to make the time in your life to enjoy the changes that begin to happen as you take care of those needs.

The Importance of Rest and Relaxation

Just as important as exercise in NS disorders are appropriate amounts of rest and relaxation. As happens so often in our lives as we're buried under the stress of unbalanced living, we forget to care lovingly for ourselves. Some of the most basic human needs, such as a loving, supportive environment, good nutrition, exercise, rest, and relaxation, are sacrificed. We look for instant cures and remedies in the drugs that are available today and dig ourselves further into the pits of our despair. But remedies are more often found in basic lifestyle changes; these are the true "medicines" that create balance and harmony.

During periods of extreme tension or NS disorders, some people find they don't sleep well. If they fall asleep, it is restless and disturbed. For others, the reverse is true; they fall into periods of deep sleep and never seem to wake up fully.

Both problems stem from a similar NS imbalance and both can be corrected with proper nutrition and natural herbal remedies. The proper amounts of rest and relaxation are extremely important for NS health and balance.

Chemicals such as seratonin are produced only during particular times of sleep and are vitally necessary for mental function. The need for sleep is not so much to rest our bodies as it is to rest our minds. The body needs little more than two hours of sleep per day to function, but parts of the brain need seven to eight hours to be fully recharged and rested. There are simple but highly effective methods that ensure that one gets more rest in times of stress. Above all, remember to:

Avoid staying up late at night. You also may wish to follow some of the suggestions under Insomnia for specific suggestions on how to ensure deep, restful sleep.

Learn to say no to extra activities, especially those in the late evening. Though they may be fun and entertaining, many of those extra activities require the very energy needed to refuel and restore a depleted nervous system. Whenever something seems really important or necessary to do, ask yourself how much energy it will require. Remind yourself that what is most important in your life at this time *is feeling really good, rested, and vital.* I think often of the Biblical story of Joseph and the coffers of grain he stored as an assurance against famine. To me, this story is a reminder of the access we have to plentiful energy. But in order for that energy to be everlasting, we must not use it all up. We must also replenish the energy we borrow from the coffers by sleeping, eating well, exercising, and striving to live lives of harmony and balance.

Flower Essences: Nature's Most Radiant Remedies

Flower essences were "discovered" and made popular by the works of the great master of healing, Dr. Edward Bach. A prominent physician in England during the early 20th century,

Bach became dissatisfied with the conventional healing modalities of modern medicine and returned to the fields of his childhood. There he discovered the healing power inherent in flowers. Devising a remarkably simple, safe, and effective system of healing from the flowers, he treated all manner of illness by addressing the emotions behind the problems. The system is brilliant in its simplicity and humbling in its effectiveness. Though the flower essences might possibly stretch one's belief in the rational world, there are thousands of recorded cases of its effectiveness in treating physical ailments.

Since Dr. Bach's death in the early '50s, many people have chosen to carry on his work with the flower essences and have developed literally thousands of flower essences for all manner of disorders. But, always and foremost, the flowers address the spirit of the illness, the underlying cause, the emotional being.

Because I am most familiar with Dr. Bach's remedies, I continue to use them. However, I am convinced that those flower essences made from North American plants have a special affinity for people who live on this continent. No matter which flower essences you choose, be sure that they are ethically prepared. The flower essences are energetic medicines working on the powerful yet subtle vibrational levels of healing; how the medicines are prepared is of utmost importance.

Flower essences are available in natural foods stores across the country. In fact, one can find flower essences in most countries in the world, a testament of their effectiveness. They are liquid extracts that can be used with any other system of healing or medication with no harmful side effects. One simply places a drop or two of the selected essence under the tongue several times a day. Flower essences are tasteless and odorless preparations. They are absorbed instantly into the system and begin their healing work seconds after ingested.

For trauma, anxiety, stress, and other NS disorders there are a number of flower essences that are particularly valuable.

A Guide to Flower Essences

FLOWER ESSENCE	USE
Aspen	Indicated for fear of the unknown, vague anxiety and apprehension, hidden fears, and nightmares
Gorse	Used for discouragement, hopelessness, and resignation
Hornbean	Indicated for fatigue, weariness, or when daily life is seen as an overwhelming burden
Impatiens	Recommended for impatience, irritation, tension, and intolerance
Mimulus	Used for known fears of everyday life and shyness
Mustard	Indicated for melancholy, gloom, despair, and general depression without obvious cause
Olive	Excellent for complete exhaustion after a long struggle
Rescue Remedy (also called Five-Flower Remedy)	The most famous of all the flower essences, this combination of five flowers is especially suited for trauma and stressful situations
Rock Rose	Suggested for deep fear, terror, panic attacks, fear of death or annihilation
Star of Bethlehem	Used for shock or trauma, either recent or from a past experience; also indicated for the need for comfort and reassurance from the spiritual world
Vervain	Recommended for nervous exhaustion from overstriving
White Chestnut	Indicated for a worrisome, chattering mind
Wild Rose	Indicated for resignation, lack of hope, or lingering illness

WOODLAND ESSENCES: A CUT ABOVE

My friends Kate Gilday and Don Babineau of Woodland Essences have been making essences from endangered plants. By gently bending the blossoms into spring water or sprinkling water over the flowers, they are able to capture the medicinal properties without injury to the plants. These exquisite remedies are already proving to be invaluable in treating rare and unusual illnesses. (See Resources for the address of Woodland Essences.)

Avoid Irritating Foods

The previous suggestions, basic though they are, are guaranteed to enhance the health of your nervous system. But if you are to achieve optimum health there are certain foods that are necessary to avoid. Rather than being redundant (most people are aware that these foods are potential troublemakers) they're listed here with a gentle reminder that, ultimately, they are really are not worth the trouble they cause.

Chocolate

Called "the food of the gods" in the languages of the people who first discovered and used it, chocolate was and is a "holy" food. Like most substances held sacred, it was not intended to be consumed often, certainly not every day. Chocolate originally was not served with sugar. In fact, it may have been considered an abomination to sweeten chocolate. It was most often mixed with other bitter herbs and spiced with a bit of hot pepper to make a delicious, spicy beverage. The original formula is, by my standards, a far more interesting and delicious drink.

Coffee and Other Caffeine-Rich Foods

Stimulants are contraindicated in most imbalances involving the nervous system. Foods high in caffeine especially are to be avoided. Not only do they overstimulate an already tired system, but they further agitate the adrenal glands, contributing to adrenal exhaustion, fatigue, and depression. Adrenal exhaustion is the root cause of many of the problems associated with the nervous system and plays a big part in depression and anxiety disorders.

Prescribed in therapeutic dosages, coffee and other caffeine-rich foods have been successfully used to ward off migraines (if taken at the early signs). They also serve as excellent "emergency energy" for situations such as late-night driving. Of course, caffeine addiction and withdrawal symptoms are a prime source of agitation for the nervous system. There are basically two methods recommended to withdraw from this most common of all addictions; one is cold turkey, the other is a gradual, steady withdrawal. See page 60 for instructions on how to give up coffee with kindness.

Processed, Refined Foods

The foods that fall into this category fill huge grocery stores and occupy most of the space on people's kitchen shelves. In a short period of history we have digressed from an almost totally natural diet dependent on the Earth's simple riches, foods that have evolved over centuries for compatibility with our genetic makeup, to a diet replete with food colorings, pesticides, synthetic hormones, and, most recently, genetically engineered foods. This chemical bath we subject our bodies to daily has taken its toll. For a complete discussion on the effects of this change in the eating patterns of our species, I direct you to two excellent books: *Nourishing Traditions* by Sally Fallon and *Healing with Whole Foods* by Paul Pitchford. If you believe that diet doesn't affect your health, follow the guidelines that Andrew Weil sets forth in *8 Weeks to Optimum Health*. If you don't feel better after eight weeks on his suggested regime, then you are one of those rare individuals who food doesn't affect.

Sugars and Sweets

Sugar in all its many forms provides quick, high-powered energy to the body. The problem is the energy is used quickly, often leaving one feeling more tired than ever. The huge sugar consumption of Americans — more than 126 pounds per person per year — may be more directly linked to the abnormally high percentage of depression, anxiety, and personality disorders experienced in the United States than we have previously thought.

Aside from providing short-term energy, sugar further depletes the nervous system by utilizing precious calcium in its digestive process. The nervous system is dependent on high levels of blood calcium in order to function at its maximum potential. Sugar competes for this calcium. No wonder you feel agitated, annoyed, or depressed after a sugar binge has worn off. The calcium levels drop as the sugar is digested, leaving irritable nerve endings.

Alcohol

Even small amounts of alcohol when one is suffering from NS disorders can be disorienting. Alcohol is often sought as a crutch during times of stress and depression, but further depresses the system. It is a highly addictive substance for some people; oddly, those who need it the least are the ones most avidly addicted to it. Alcohol addiction — as with addiction of any kind — is challenging at best, and devastating at worst. It's difficult to recover from its grips without personal loss and an iron-clad will.

Alcohol, like sugar, demands calcium in its digestive process, thus leaching the nervous system of valuable nutrients. When suffering from NS imbalances, it is best to avoid alcohol altogether, or to drink only moderate amounts. If there is a tendency toward alcohol sensitivity, depression, anxiety, or panic attacks, avoid alcohol as if your life depended on it. It might. Don't use alcohol-based tinctures. Instead, use tinctures made from glycerin or vinegar, or take your herbs in capsules and tea instead.

Recommended Reading

Herbs are such multifaceted personalities, no one book will provide all there is to know about a plant. My suggestion is to select at least three good titles on the subject, more if possible, and keep these handy for referencing each herb when you're first introduced to it. Just like it's best to use more than one expert for advice, it is important to glean information from more than one book. Following are some of my favorite books on herbal medicine:

Buhner, Stephen. *Sacred Plant Medicine.* Boulder, CO: Roberts Rhinehart Publishers, 1996.

Chevallier, Andrew. *The Encyclopedia of Medicinal Plants.* New York: DK Publishing, 1996.

Cowen, Eliot. *Plant Spirit Medicine.* Newberg. OR: Swan, Raven & Company, 1995.

de Baircli Levy, Juliette. *Common Herbs for Natural Health.* Woodstock, NY: Ash Tree, 1997.

———. *Traveler's Joy.* Woodstock, NY: Ash Tree, 1997.

Gladstar, Rosemary. *Herbal Healing for Women.* New York: Simon & Schuster, 1993.

Hobbs, Christopher. *The Foundations of Herbalism.* Capitola, CA: Botanica Press, 1992.

———. *Herbal Remedies for Dummies.* New York: IDG Books, 1998.

Hoffman, David. *The New Holistic Herbal.* Rockport, MA: Element Books, 1993.

Keville, Kathie. *Herbs for Health and Healing.* Emmaus, PA: Rodale Press, 1996.

Pedersen, Mark. *Nutritional Herbology.* Warsaw, IN: Wendell Whitman Co., 1994.

Sturdivant, Lee, and Tim Blakley. *Medicinal Herbs in the Garden, Field, and Marketplace.* Friday Harbor, WA: San Juan Naturals, 1998.

Tilford, Gregory. *From Earth to Herbalist.* Missoula, MT: Mountain Press, 1998.

Wardwell, Joyce. *The Herbal Home Remedy Book.* Pownal, VT: Storey Communications, 1998.

Wood, Matthew. *The Book of Herbal Wisdom.* Berkeley, CA: North Atlantic Books, 1998.

Resources

Where to Find Herbs

Thankfully, herbs and herbal products are now widely available. I generally suggest purchasing herbal products from local sources, as it helps support bioregional herbalism and community-based herbalists. However, here are some of my favorite sources for high-quaility herbs and herbal products.

Frontier Herbs

P.O. Box 299
Norway, IA 52318
(800) 669-3275
Aside from having an incredible list of supplies and herbs, Frontier empha-sizes medicinal plant con-servation and preservation. Frontier is a wholesale sup-plier, but offers price breaks for individual buyers.

Green Mountain Herbs

P.O. Box 532
Putney, VT 05436
(888) 4GRNMTS

Healing Spirits

9198 State Route 415
Avoca, NY 14809
(607) 566-2701
One of the best sources of ethically wildcrafted and organically grown herbs in the Northeast.

Jean's Greens

119 Sulphur Springs Road
Newport, NY 13146
(315) 845-6500
A wonderful selection of fresh and dried organic and wildcrafted herbs. Also, oils, containers, beeswax, and other materials needed for making herbal products.

Mountain Rose

20818 High Street
North San Juan, CA 95960
(800) 879-3337
A small herb company nes-tled in the coastal moun-tains of northern California, Mountain Rose supplies bulk herbs, beeswax, books, oils, and containers.

Trinity Herbs
P.O. Box 1001
Graton, CA 95444
(707) 824-2040
Trinity is a small wholesale herb company that sells bulk herbs in quantities of one pound or more.

Wild Weeds
1302 Camp Wcott Road
Ferndale, CA 95536
(800) 553-9453
A small herbal emporium, this mail-order business was initially started to supply correspondence-course students with the herbs and herbal materials they needed.

Woodland Essences
PO Box 206
Cold Brook, NY 13324
(315) 845-1515

Handmade Herbal Products

Each of the following companies provides high-quality herbal products. Write for their current catalogs and price lists.

Avena Botanicals
20 Mill Street
Rockland, ME 04841

Empowered Herbals
3481 Myers Lane
St. James City, FL 33956
Try their excellent drink made from spirulina.

Equinox Botanicals
33446 McCumber Road
Rutland, OH 45775

Green Terrestrial
P.O. Box 266
Milton, NY 12547

Herb Pharm
Box 116
Williams, OR 97544

Herbalists and Alchemists
P.O. Box 553
Broadway, NJ 08808

Sage Mountain Herb Products
General Delivery
Lake Elmore, VT 05657
(802) 888-7278
Rosemary Gladstar's company.

Simpler's Botanicals
P.O. Box 39
Forestville, CA 95436

Zand Herbal Products
Products available in most natural foods and herb stores across the country.

Educational Resources

A few years ago it was difficult to find herbal educational opportunities, but today the choices are many. Following are a few well-known herbal schools and programs.

American Herb Association (AHA)
P.O. Box 1673
Nevada City, CA 95959
More complete listings of schools, programs, seminars, and correspondence courses offered throughout the United States. There is a small fee for this publication.

American Herbalist Guild (AHG)
Box 746555
Arvada, CO 80006
More complete listings of schools, programs, seminars, and correspondence courses offered throughout the United States. There is a small fee for this publication.

The California School of Herbal Studies
P.O. Box 39
Forestville, CA 95476
One of the oldest and most respected herb schools in the United States, founded by Rosemary Gladstar in 1982.

Herb Research Foundation
1007 Pearl Street, Suite 200
Boulder, CO 80302
This is simply the best herbal resource and research facility in America. They also have a newsletter.

The Northeast Herb Association
P.O. Box 10
Newport, NY 13416

Rocky Mountain Center for Botanical Studies
1705 Fourteenth Street, #287
Boulder, CO 80302
Offers excellent programs for beginners, as well as advanced clinical training programs.

Sage Mountain Retreat Center and Botanical Sanctuary
P.O. Box 420
East Barre, VT 05649
Apprentice programs and classes with Rosemary Gladstar and other well-known herbalists.

The Science and Art of Herbalism: A Home Study Course
by Rosemary Gladstar
P.O. Box 420
East Barre, VT 05649
The Science and Art of Herbalism was written in an inspiring and joyful manner for students wishing a systematic, in-depth study of herbs. The course emphasizes the foundations of herbalism, wildcrafting, Earth awareness, and herbal preparation and formulation. The heart of the course is the development of a deep personal relationship with the plant world.

Herb Newsletters

The American Herb Association Newsletter
P.O. Box 1673
Nevada City, CA 95959

Business of Herbs
North Winds Farm
439 Pondersona Way
Jemez Springs, NM 87025

Foster's Botanical and Herb Reviews
P.O. Box 106
Eureka Springs, AR 72632

HerbalGram
P.O. Box 201660
Austin, TX 78720

The Herb Quarterly
P.O. Box 548
Boiling Springs, PA 17007

Herbs for Health and *The Herb Companion*
201 East Fourth Street
Loveland, CO 80537

Medical Herbalism
P.O. Box 33080
Portland, OR 97233

Planetary Formula Newsletter
c/o Roy Upton
P.O. Box 533
Soquel, CA 95073

United Plant Savers
P.O. Box 420
East Barre, VT 05649

Wild Foods Forum
4 Carlisle Way NE
Atlanta, GA 30308

United Plant Savers At-Risk List

United Plant Savers (UpS) is a nonprofit, grassroots organization dedicated to preserving native American medicinal plants and the land that they grow on. An organization for herbalists and people who love and use plants, our purpose is to ensure the future of our rich diversity of medicinal plants through organic cultivation, sustainable wildcrafting practices, creating botanical sanctuaries for medicinal plant conservation, and reestablishing native plant communities in their natural environments.

The following herbs have been designated as "UpS At Risk" due to overharvesting, loss of habitat, or by nature of their innate rareness or sensitivity. UpS is not asking for a moratorium on the use of these herbs, but rather is asking for a concerted effort by all those who use plants as medicine to seek sustainable alternatives; that is, grow your own, buy from reputable companies, or substitute other herbs whenever possible.

American Ginseng *(Panax quinquefolius)*

Black Cohosh *(Cimicifuga racemosa)*

Bloodroot *(Sanguinaria canadensis)*

Blue Cohosh *(Caulophyllum thalictroides)*

Echinacea (*Echinacea* species)

Goldenseal *(Hydrastis canadensis)*

Helonias Root *(Chamaelirium luteum)*

Kava Kava *(Piper methysticum)* (Hawaii only)

Lady's-Slipper (*Cypripedium* species)

Lomatium *(Lomatium dissectum)*

Osha (*Ligusticum porteri* and related species)

Partridgeberry *(Mitchella repens)*

Peyote *(Lophophora williamsii)*

Slippery elm *(Ulmus rubra)*

Sundew (*Drosera* species)

Trillium, Beth root (*Trillium* species)

True Unicorn *(Aletris farinosa)*

Venus's-flytrap *(Dionaea muscipula)*

Wild Yam (*Dioscorea villosa* and related species)

For more information on United Plant Savers and how you can become involved in "Planting the Future," contact United Plant Savers, P.O. Box 98, East Barre, VT 05649; (802) 479-9825; E-mail: info@www.plantsavers.org.

Index

Other Storey Books You Will Enjoy

Also in the Rosemary Gladstar series: *Herbal Remedies for Children's Health,* ISBN 1-58017-153-2; *Herbal Remedies for Men's Health,* ISBN 1-58017-151-6; *Herbs for Longevity and Well-Being,* ISBN 1-58017-154-0; *Herbs for Natural Beauty,* ISBN 1-58017-152-4; and *Herbs for the Home Medicine Chest,* ISBN 1-58017-156-7.

Healing with Herbs, by Penelope Ody. This visual introduction to the world of herbal medicine offers clear, illustrated instructions for growing, preparing, and administering healing herbs to relieve a variety of ailments. 160 pages. Hardcover. ISBN 1-58017-144-3.

Herbal Antibiotics, by Stephen Harrod Buhner. This book presents all the current information about antibiotic-resistant microbes and the herbs that are most effective in fighting them. Readers will also find detailed, step-by-step instructions for making and using herbal infusions, tinctures, teas, and salves to treat various types of infections. 128 pages. Paperback. ISBN 1-58017-148-6.

The Herbal Home Remedy Book, by Joyce A. Wardwell. Discover how to use 25 common herbs to make simple herbal remedies. Native American legends and folk-lore are spread throughout the book. 176 pages. Paperback. ISBN 1-58017-016-1.

Herbal Remedy Gardens, by Dorie Byers. An introduction to more than 20 herbs, their medicinal uses, propagation, and harvesting techniques, this book includes dozens of easy-to-make recipes for common ailments. Thirty-eight illustrated garden plans offer choices for customizing a garden to fit your special health needs. 224 pages. Paperback. ISBN 1-58017-095-1.

Herbal Tea Gardens, by Marietta Marshall Marcin. This tea lover's gardening bible contains full instructions for growing and brewing tea herbs, plus more than 100 recipes that make use of their healthful qualities. Readers will find complete plans for customized gardens suitable for plots or containers. 192 pages. ISBN 1-58017-106-0.

Making Herbal Dream Pillows, by Jim Long. In this lavishly illustrated book, you'll find step-by-step instructions for creating 15 herbal dream blends and pillows for custom-made dreams. Author Jim Long also explores the history of dream pillows and their ties to folk medicine and herbal mythology. 64 pages. Hardcover. ISBN 1-58017-075-7.

These and other Storey Books are available at your bookstore, farm store, garden center, or directly from Storey Books, Schoolhouse Road, Pownal, Vermont 05261, or by calling 1-800-441-5700. Or visit our Web site at www.storey.com.